A
Token of Love
for Your Body's Health
and Beauty

A
Token of Love
for Your Body's Health
and Beauty

Practical guides to improve your appearance and fitness

A. M. ZAIN

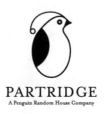

PARTRIDGE

A Penguin Random House Company

To order additional copies of this book, contact
Toll Free 800 101 2657 (Singapore)
Toll Free 1 800 81 7340 (Malaysia)
orders.singapore@partridgepublishing.com

www.partridgepublishing.com/singapore

Dedicated to Surya K., and Z. Hamid

PREFACE

We live in complex environment with the cosmopolitan people dynamically changes due to industrialization, urbanization and technology advancement move according to global market demand that influence the socio-economic, environment and peoples attributes. Nowadays, success is defined by the economic stability and prosperity while quite often overlook the healthy living, social need and environment sustainability. Majority of population suffers from pollution, ecosystem imbalance and extreme conditions. As consequence effect, the emergence of new diseases spread in certain areas cause health threats to people. Added more stress to the public besides the current challenge. Personal health care sometimes is forgotten due to high demanding tasks. The personal health care is inculcates through daily practice. Simple health practices and body fitness techniques to enhance health and beauty is described in this book. Healthy body is developed by taking a balance nutrient. The intake of food rich in antioxidant together with regular exercises will help you maintain your fitness. Your good habits will be fruitful at the ends of day which will greatly improve your body's mind and spirit. This will shape the inner shine natural beauty from a healthy body. It is individual preference for taking cares of your own asset, but with essential knowledge of real practice and awareness, it can motivate you in developing a balance and harmony life. This book is dedicated for all who is looking for guidance in coping with complex life and busy days while maintaining healthy living. It is compilation of life experience and healthcare gathered by different aspect and angle from inherited believes blend with science fact and figures. The balance of all facet of life is considered to bring the optimum healthy living of human being physically and mentally. From inside soul to the outside of human body fitness and find the best matches in all that can save your journey from harmful life interferences.

ACKNOWLEDGEMENT

I would like to express my sincere appreciation to my parents for provide me with the best childhood moment with utmost love and attention. I feel very fortunate to have all of family members stay in united and very passionate in giving the moral and materials supports for the preparation of the manuscripts. Special appreciation to my hubby for the cooperation and understanding in providing the quality time on the write-up, day and night in conducing environment which make this book viable. I would like to thank to all friends and colleagues who have helped me during my hard time and good time for being as supportive and helpful. Your contributions to my knowledge gain and improvement shaped my current success. The lesson learnt from our mother nature with all great happening curves the beautiful life experience during this journey to eternity. My deep gratitude expression for the blessing and meaningful precious gifts from God the Almighty in facing the life challenges. Thank you for being very supportive, passionate and cares.

CONTENTS

Preface..vii
Acknowledgement...ix
List of Figures...xiv
List of Tables..xiv
List of Abbreviation..xv

1.0   Healthy Mind and Body..1
      1.1 Health Challenge...2
      1.2 Modern Lifestyle...3

2.0   Health Traps around Us...7
      2.1 Commonly Affected Diseases...7
            2.1.1 Hepatitis...7
            2.1.2 HIV/AIDS..8
            2.1.3 Influenza..8
            2.1.4 Malaria...8
      2.2 The Deadly Diseases...9
      2.3 Non-Communicable Diseases..10
      2.4 Occupational Diseases..11

3.0   Monitoring the Health Condition...13
      3.1 Blood Pressure...13
      3.2 Glucose Level...14
      3.3 Body Mass Index...15
      3.4 Tongue Discoloration..15

4.0   Cosmetic and Skincare..17
      4.1 Harmful Additives...17
      4.2 Create Your Own Cosmetic...19

5.0   Nutrients for Health Maintenance..21
      5.1 Recommended Daily Allowance...21
      5.2 Food for Thought...22
      5.3 Brain Damaging Habits and How to Optimize Brain Functionality.....23
      5.4 Elements in Our Body..24

6.0   Health Inhibitors 27
      6.1 Stress Development 28
      6.2 Stress Relieves Methods 29

7.0   Tip to Stay Away from Chronic Diseases 33
      7.1 Balancing Vital Components 33
      7.2 Top 5 Fruits for Antioxidants 37
      7.3 Obesity Effect to Health and Images 38
      7.4 Techniques on How to Prevent Cancer 40
            7.4.1 Dairies products 40
            7.4.2 Vitamin D 40
            7.4.3 Plastic polymer 40
            7.4.4 Health awareness 41
            7.4.5 De-stress activity 41

8.0   Simple Steps for Body Fitness and Beauty 43
      8.1 Tai Chi 43
      8.2 Eskay Technique 44
      8.3 Reflexology 44
      8.4 Rejuvenation Tips for Reverse Aging 44
      8.5 How to Boost Flawless Skin 46

9.0   Beautiful Figure Practices 47
      9.1 Facelift 47
      9.2 Breathing Practice 48
      9.3 Toning Muscles 49
      9.4 Remove Fat and Double Chin Layer 50
      9.5 Tuning and Tightening Bust Shape 51
      9.6 Cellulite 51
      9.7 Flabby Arms 51

10.0 Reveling the Healthy Diet 53
      10.1 Antioxidants 53
      10.2 Immediate Remedy for Common Health Problem 56
      10.3 Eating for Health 58

11.0 Vital Organ for Beautiful Blossom 61
      11.1 Kidney for Liquidity Filtration 61
      11.2 Liver for all the Good Senses 61
      11.3 Heart the Key for Life Survivor 62

12.0   Synergizing the Body's Energy 65
    12.1 Energy House...65
    12.2 Mental Energy 65
        12.2.1 Brain waves 66
        12.2.2 Brain booster 67
    12.3 Heart Energy 67
    12.4 Gen 2 Energy 68

References...69

LIST OF FIGURES

Figure 1 Life risks and protection factors
Figure 2 The tongue map
Figure 3 Sources of oxygen deficient
Figure 4 Fruits rich in antioxidants, avocado and grapefruit
Figure 5 Antibiotic points on upper part of the foot, A, B and C
Figure 6 Left foot reflexology points
Figure 7 Face-lift to reduce the wrinkle and strengthening face muscles
Figure 8 Toning and tightening the (a) buttock (b) thigh (c) waistline and (d) stomach muscles
Figure 9 *Carica papaya* leaves useful for the treatment of fever and rejuvenation
Figure 10 *Androghapis paniculata* shrubs for the treatment of diabetes mellitus

LIST OF TABLES

Table 1 Blood pressure in mm Hg
Table 2 Pre-meal blood glucose
Table 3 BMI Categories (NIH, 2015)
Table 4 Tongue discoloration and associated illness or body conditions
Table 5 RDA Vitamin and minerals for adults
Table 6 Cholesterol content in variety of multi food sources (MSD)
Table 7 Activity factor to account for BMR
Table 8 Plant sources of antioxidants
Table 9 Key food for each phase of life
Table 10 Healthy fruit juice blends for body improvement

LIST OF ABBREVIATION

AIDS	Acquired immunodeficiency syndrome
ALA	Alpha lipoic acid
BMI	Body Mass Index
BMR	Basal metabolic rate
BPA	Bisphenol A
CAE	Carboxyl alkyl esters
CFR	Glomeruler filtration rate
CKD	Chronic kidney disease
CVD	Cardiovascular disease
DEA	Diethanolamine
DHA	Docosahexaenoic acid
DNA	Deoxynuclic acid
EFAs	Essential fatty acids
EFT	Emotional freedom technique
EPA	Eicosapentaenoic acid
FCC	Federal Communication Commission
FOS	Fructo-oligosaccharides
GABA	Gamma amino butyric acid
GI	Glycemic Index
GLA	Gamma-linolenic acid
H1N1	Haemagglutinin 1 Neuraminidase 1
HDL	High-density lipoprotein
HIV	Human immunodeficiency virus
IGF-1	Insulin Growth Factor 1
IR	Infra-red
LDL	Low-density lipoprotein
MERS-CoV	Middle east respiratory syndrome-corona virus

MSG	Monosodium glutamines
NCD	Non-communicable disease
ORAC	Oxygen radical absorbance capacity
PMS	Premenstrual syndrome
RDA	Recommended Daily Allowance
ROS	Reactive oxygen species
SAR	Specific absorption rate
SARs	Severe acute respiratory syndrome
SOD	Superoxide dismutases
SPF	Skin Protection filter
TEA	Triethanolamin
THMs	Trihalomethanes
UV-A / B	Ultra violet A / B
WHO	World Health Organization

Chapter 1

Healthy Mind and Body

All of us are familiar with the two most important words for the ambitious moderate man on the earth reaching the dream of an ideal life, health and beauty. Well the third one of course wealth. If one's have all the three means the life is in their hand. Health and beauty are independence i.e. if you have beautiful figurine not necessary mean you are healthy. But if you are beautiful and healthy, then the wealth is part of yours as wealth is the possession of material including your health and body. Healthy body and mind are the great gift in one's life. But how many of us know how to stay in healthy condition and maintained the life until the end of day.

Stay in healthy condition means a state of complete physical, mental, and social wellbeing not merely the absence of diseases and infirmity or defect. The effort to stay in a healthy state comes with knowledge and practice of a healthy lifestyle. The healthy body, mind and spirit are the result of living in harmony within population and the environment, regular body maintenance and well-adapted to dynamic complex socio-economic populations.

This book share with you handy healthy tips and practices observed from different group of ethnics, cultures and regions from traditional to moderns daily life. Essential and practical habits can somehow save your days for consulting medical doctors and relieved the dependents on prescribed medicines. The state of being healthy also provides you with the advantage of extra money save from spending on medical bills and consultation fees. It is great beneficial to learn from many ancient practices for you own goodness. The proven effective natures healing from the environment with abundant materials available for us are stored with hidden benefit for maintaining the health and beauty for those who cares.

1.1 HEALTH CHALLENGE

Healthy means you have not been infected by any chronic disease, with mental and physical fitness for performing conventional task and ride the life journey with agility and endurance. Mental fitness allows you to think and behave as per acceptable norm and ethics in the communities. The burdens to mental health may accelerate the schizophrenia, depression, epilepsy, dementia, alcohol dependence, neurological and substance-use disorder cases.

Physical fitness is the capacity to perform all assigned task and duties as per intended functional procedure. Lacks of physical fitness can cause work delays, frequent medical leaves and additional cost for treatment. At the end the lack of physical fitness ripple effect move toward management structure, operation and maintenance, and performance quality of the stakeholder or employer thus also determine the revenue.

There are strong relationship of spiritual believes with the physical fitness. The moment you understand the relationship, it will open you to tap the benefit of all materials in the universe to provide you with all your needs.

Staying in the highly competence world has put stress to the public peoples. The stress level developed gradually which can easily affect the human behavior and body response to the stress factor is indicates by the symptoms of:

1. Show aggressive behaviors toward minor error or conflicts with expression of anger, impatient, grueling and dangerous actions
2. Additive to alcohol, drug, coffee or tobacco
3. Consume additional food or loss appetite
4. Insomnia or sleep disabilities
5. Reduced focus at work and performance efficiency
6. Easily fall into sickness as stress weaken body's immune system

Stress has good impact if the person received stress with positive outlook. The stress can motivate the receiver to work out of the box or harder and at the same time induce the hormonal system ready to fight the current situation or overcome the conflict in different ways. Problem associated with the stress factor must be critically scrutinize and analyzed for potential solution. The clever action is to do holistic review or 'seeing the battlefield' and provides strategy for facing the problem.

Consider all aspects in the current challenge, the advantages, disadvantages, loss and gain and then determine or looking at your goal and target. The roles of each person around you may give certain influence toward your actions, but remember you are the boss of your own activity. You are the key player in your own life, move your ball toward your targeted direction.

Safeguard your life from harmful effects through right knowledge and physical fitness. Consume all the vital nutrients to nourish your body, promote the good feeling by following useful health activities such as learning the Yoga and Tai-Chi, practiced to moderate your anger and anxiety through socializing, listening to soothing sound, try to have regular deep relaxation to release stress and learned new thing if you have free time to activate the mind, to stay in connected and excited mood.

Meditation or pray is good ways to harmonize the body system, clear mind and uplift the spirit, so your body is synchronize in alpha waves. The waves that can help you solving the problem clear your sight and stay in peace with the natures around you. The alpha wave can be used to help you achieved your target which should be played before bedtimes. Just remember your target and make affirmation of you goal before you fall asleep. It is one of the effective ways to attract your goal become reality. The affirmation of your goal can motivate successful achievement sometimes faster than you expected.

If you are trap in acute situation, remember your body has intrinsic power to remedy itself. Just listen to the body's need, where actually your body can talk, by gut feeling and you are doing good thing to be in better state. Our cell is intelligent enough to tell your brain for immediate response to cope and adapt to the problem, either during emergency or in daily life threat situation.

1.2 MODERN LIFESTYLE

We live in modern lifestyle with rapid change in technology and IT gadgets for fast and easy operations and communications. All of these instruments and apparatus help in handling routine and tedious works at home and office becomes necessary items for human need. But all new inventions and gadgets which greatly improved repeated task, solve complex systems or integrated or simplify communication are associated with hidden or inherent risks.

The limitation in working conditions and how we manage critical situation and problem arise during assigned work may generate stress. The stress management must be acquired to minimize the health impact. The awareness of healthy lifestyle and safe habit must be inculcated at workplace as well as to the public. Excessive stress may lead to mental disability to perform it intended function.

Unhealthy lifestyle and development of diseases are closely connected explained why so many people caught into heart attack, diabetes, poisoning, obesity, high blood pressure and virus infection. The affected person received or developed the diseases through their polluted environment, from inhalation of chemical or biological agents either airborne, waterborne or upon direct body contact with the virus or bacteria. The combination of non-communicable diseases with the communicable diseases may create a complexity of infections to the modern societies.

The emergence of new viral infection from the working grounds or remote areas to the public peoples forming breaking news lately from so called deadly disease of Ebola, SARs, HINI which become epidemic in certain region caused restriction on utilization, export of specific products or migration of peoples from or to infected areas.

We have to adapt our life to the complex technology developed without complete understanding of its impacts and consequence. Hand phone utilization has a direct impact causing hotspot in brain from the wave radiation measured as specific absorption rate (SAR) in watt/kg. The SAR was controlled below 1.6 watt/kg by Federal Communication Commission (FCC). The higher SAR received by the brain from hand phone antenna may cause brain cancer.

Home cooking by microwave has advantage of fast and easy cooking but most of the scientist and experts did not use the microwave for everyday cooking due to it long term impact to internal human body was still in ambiguous states. The ways microwave changes matter was still questionable. The usage of plastics containers is definitely not advisable for microwave cooking as plastics are easily degraded.

The latest trend in the beauty practice is moving toward beautiful skin and youthful appearance. Many of us just purchase a well claimed skincare products for fairer skin and delay the aging signs without concerning about the sources of their skincare products.

In order to prepare a skincare product, the producer use the same nutrients derived from food varieties for consumption and this condition will put pressure on cost of corps production. The available food for consumption become scarce as there are group of people ready to pay high prices for cosmetic and skin cares products, and we see at the end certain food such as fruit becomes expensive.

We have to remember that each of us is already safeguard by a well-covered melanin layer to protect unnecessary ray. Any attempt to remove the natural protection cell, for a fairer skin, will expose internal epidermis and dermis layers to harmful radiation of UV-A and UV-B rays from sunlight.

Longer waves of UV-A in the range of 320-400 nm is dormant tanning ray which can penetrate deeper into the skin surface causing skin aging and wrinkle. This ray can penetrate glass material while UV-B cannot penetrate the solid glass.

The UV-B ray, found in shorter range of 290-320 nm is intensified during 10 am to 4 pm can cause burn and damage to the skin. The UV-B exposures create premature ageing, cataracts and cancer. It is advisable to protect skin using multi spectrum sunscreen, such as zinc oxide to protect from both rays.

Minimum sun protection factor, SPF 15 is recommended by Skin Cancer Foundation which can filter 93 % of the UV-B. Most of the sun block and day cream are already designed with the SPF 15, SPF 25 or SPF 50 to protect skin according to individual requirement.

Every day we are exposed to so many risk factors from the contaminated food, traffic conditions, hazardous chemicals, haze, radiations, extreme heat and pressure, infectious agents, and social problems.

The risks in life journey begin from the birth time to the old age are link to the parent's genetic, environment and occupation which should be safeguarded by the protection factors including the healthy parent's genetic and parental cares, knowledge on health awareness, ethical behavior and attitude, health care and social support.

Figure 1 depicts the life risks and protection factors in life journey. The risk may increase with the age due to nature of human being activity, larger responsibility, accountability and physical fitness degradation.

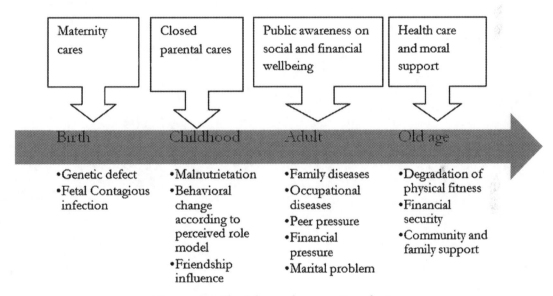

Figure 1: Life risks and protection factors

Practically we do measure the risk from occupational risk or the workplace hazards, but rarely measure the whole risk in your life journey. This was due to complex life face per individual as life experience differ from one to another, in form of ethnic, culture, food, geography, lifestyle and climate.

But there are similarities in the human being, we are affected by the same microorganism attacks, we have quite the same plant species, we move around and meet each other as a socialized groups, we are affected by the same diseases, our objectives in life is almost the same to achieve the successful life and prevent all the unpleasant things from enter into our life.

CHAPTER 2
HEALTH TRAPS AROUND US

2.1 COMMONLY AFFECTED DISEASES

We live in an open globe and share the raw material with other kingdoms including the animals, plant, virus and bacteria which will expose us to communicable diseases, easily spread from one to another or from animal to people. The spread of communicable diseases occurs via airborne and waterborne or through blood or body fluid contact or secretion. The terms infectious and contagious are also used to describe communicable disease. We have to learn about coordinated efforts to combat current communicable diseases and prevent the spread which know no boundaries.

2.1.1 Hepatitis

Viral hepatitis causes 78% of liver cancers and the hepatitis B virus alone infects an estimated one in three people worldwide. The public health concern of viral hepatitis is growing as the viruses are easily transmitted from person to person. The spread of viral disease is prevented through the use of clean water and food. Hepatitis B can migrate to new patient through food prepared by person with hepatitis B. The safer way to reduce hepatitis infection through body's contact is to cook your own food. Reduce eating in public areas if the environment is apparently unhealthy.

Try to reduce the uses of congested space like public train, bus and plane where the space is shared for long hours during the journey. Infected person carrying the virus classified as air borne diseases can easily spread to other passenger through respiration system during the transfer routes.

2.1.2 HIV/AIDS

A total of 1.8 million people died from AIDS-related causes in 2009 (UNAIDS, 2011). HIV epidemic affected population in megacities due mainly to the unsafe heterosexual or homosexual exposures, drug usage or blood transmission. The virus is spread through the transfer of body fluid contact such as blood, semen and milk. The virus infects the human immune system by decrease the CD4$^+$ cells and exposed body to other infections. Prevention program to control HIV prevalence is by educate population about the infection root and safe prevention measures in dealing with the affected patients. The most successful programs to fight AIDS have been efforts to make available antiretroviral drugs that allow people with HIV to live for many years before developing symptoms of AIDS.

2.1.3 Influenza

Because influenza affects so many people around the globe every year, extensive international coordination is required in the areas of influenza surveillance, detection, and response. The influenza A (H1N1) strains virus are endemic in human being. The animal strains from pigs and birds known as swine influenza and avian influenza are also endemic. But in 2009 until 2010 the outbreak of new swine flu strain which had caused 17,000 deaths was declared as pandemic by WHO. The infected virus migrates from pig to human, but the virus may also transfer from human to human which indicate by the fever, sore throat, headache, cough and discomfort.

2.1.4 Malaria

The focus areas involved in combating malaria include public health information, science and research, prevention and control, case management, and regulating diagnostic tests and vaccines. Malaria present in almost 100 countries and threatens half of the world's population, WHO organisation's latest estimates suggest 207 million people were infected with malaria in 2012, with about 627,000 deaths, mostly in children under five years old. The disease is caused by single cell parasite transmitted through the anopheles mosquito's bite is both preventable and treatable. The symptoms of infection are headache, fatigue, nausea, fever and sweating followed by drop in child's body temperature.

Maintaining environmental cleanliness is vital to prevent the fatal outbreak caused by poor maintenance system, poor waste management in congested areas. The malaria cases affected by Plasmodium genus is greatly reduced due to the well establish prevention methods applied in many countries. The incident number reduced to 4725 in 2012 compared to 12705 in 2000 (MOH, 2014). The anti-malaria drug used to treat the virus effects are amodiaquine, chloroquine, mefloquine, quinine and sulfadoxine-pyrimethamine. The mutation and genetic change as a result of exposure to synthetic chemical dose from all kind of materials designated to improve production, increase quality and appearance has it impact to the tiny creatures that we underestimate of it capacity in returning the cycle back to human being.

The well structure urbanization in big cities requires a proper plan to manage all this issues. It is the responsibilities of all citizens who occupied the space to ensure their home is well maintained. It is not only the functions of government bodies, private organization, contractor and workers, but if the occupier negligence to maintain the cleanliness of their own space the problem still remain.

2.2 THE DEADLY DISEASES

Many deadly diseases occurred in specific areas but easily spread to other regions that cause global health threat. One of the diseases known as Ebola virus spread in West Africa has killed 10,000 people in nine countries which started in late 2013 is considered as one of deadly diseases. Infection occurs through body fluid contact with the symptom of fever, muscle pain, headache, and sore throat with the consequence effect of diarrhea, vomiting, rash, impaired kidney and liver and bleeding.

Another outbreak disease generated by SARs virus was first spotted in China went on to infect more than 8,000 people and kill more than 750 people. SARs caused sufferers to run a fever, have flu-like symptoms and have difficulty breathing. Currently, there is no known cure or vaccine for SARs. Different virus spread from camel fluid shows quite similar effects like SARs, the MERS-CoV in Saudi Arabia and Jordan in 2012 which cause pneumonia and kidney failure at severe level of infection. Even though infection on human is only 172 people and the death number of 27 but the potential of the virus to be spread across border and ocean was quite alarming seem infection was found in North Korea and Thailand.

Dengue outbreak in the tropic region lately had caused alarming impacts which already effect death tolls of about few hundred people in Malaysia from virus attack in *Aedes aegypti* or *albofictos* mosquito's bite. The mosquito's breeding grounds are found in poorly maintained drainage system residential area, commercial shop lots and construction sites where small water container like plastic bottles and cans trapped water as breeding medium. The symptoms of dengue fever in the affected patients are sickness to bone, muscle, ligament and eyes with acute fever. May cause red spot on skin, bleeding below skin surface, nose or gum followed by headache, loss appetites, diarrhoea and stomach ache.

The recorded dengue case for the first six months in 2015 is 57,180 with 162 deaths. The outbreak may be related to the flooding impact faced by many tropic regions in hot climate countries during monsoon season where wetted areas are easily available as breeding ground for mosquitoes.

2.3 NON-COMMUNICABLE DISEASES

The non-communicable disease (NCD) has affected the death of 16 million world populations each year usually in form of chronic diseases such as heart disease, stroke, cancer and diabetes according to WHO report. The NCD is related to unhealthy lifestyle which are costly and but preventable if the active lifestyle in the population is promoted. Seven of the top 10 causes of death in 2010 were chronic diseases.

Chronic diseases may be developed slowly without any symptom. Many inherited diseases are controllable if enough prevention steps plus healthy lifestyle is in practice. The identified goals in facing chronic diseases challenges are (a) public awareness (b) enhance economic, legal and environmental policies (c) modify risk factors (d) engage businesses and community (e) mitigate health impacts of poverty and urbanization and (f) reorientate health systems (Daar et al, 2007).

One of the alarming NCDs due to metabolic disorder, Diabetic Mellitus already affected 382 million of the world population in 2013 (Guriguata et al., 2014) which is escalated by the obesity. The use of processed food, malnutrition and toxicological effect of the harmful contaminant may cause complex metabolic disorder. The diabetic patient may have developed complications of high blood sugar (hyperglycemia) or low blood sugar (hypoglycemia), cardiovascular diseases especially stroke and coronary artery disease, peripheral vascular disease with gangrene in legs and feet, kidney failure and blindness at the later stage.

NCD is long term or lifetime health effects which require continuous support and prescribed medicines. Affected patients can be controlled or healed by changes in the lifestyle during the early stage. The diabetes mellitus refers to the weakness of the pancreas to produce enough insulin to regulate the blood sugar (Type 2) or failure to produce insulin (Type 1). The symptoms of Diabetes Mellitus Type 2 are fatigue, excess thirst, frequent urination, deterioration of vision.

The NCD like diabetes, cancer and stoke also known as aging diseases as the tendency to affect the older aged people is higher compared to younger groups. The risk of stroke effects on women slightly differs compared to men as women take the birth control pills and face pregnancy, miscarriage and menopause state where the situation trigger or increase rate of the blood clots.

2.4 OCCUPATIONAL DISEASES

Occupation diseases are developed from the exposure to workplace hazards which classified as:

1. Physical hazards such as heat, extreme temperature or pressure, loud noise and vibration and radiations.
2. Chemical hazards from solvent, resins, polymers, drug, fertilizer and paints
3. Ergonomic hazards design error, repeated jobs, awkward position and excessive movement
4. Biological hazards from virus, bacteria, mucus, mold or animals.
5. Psychosocial hazards from the overload, overstretch, stress and remote workstation,

Occupational diseases occur when workers are exposed to either hazardous agents or unhealthy conditions during performing jobs at work place. The contaminants from the work place activities may enter into worker's body through inhalation, body contact, injection or ingestion of contaminated air, water or food. The dust particles from silica and asbestos may cause silicosis or asbestosis especially found in construction and factory fields.

Occupational diseases may also develop from ergonomic factor where the interaction of man and machine or working platform was not properly designed with the outcome of awkward sitting or standing position while performing repeated task. As a result, discomfort to specific joint or ligament will forms tendonitis, a musculoskeletal disorder.

The prolong use of a personal computer at workplace or home can cause fatigue and strain eyes as the retina focus to short distance images, it is advise to have frequent break of every 20 minutes after facing the virtual display unit to maintain the healthy eyes and prevent from cataracts, or blindness. It is good practice to rest in a room without many electrical appliances or stay away from electric cables since the current may influence the health conditions.

The close ventilation is not good for long term health as the contaminants trap inside the room can accumulate and worker exposed to such contaminants may develop chronic diseases. The environment with limited accessed or confined space may accumulate harmful contaminants like radiation of radon, toxic vapor and dust will adversely affect the respiratory system due to lack of oxygen which may lead to asphyxiation or sudden death.

If you fall into sickness or infected by diseases, your body need to have enough rest for recovery and healing process. Don't force yourself to work during sickness and recovery period. It is normal to observe the patients eat less than normal quantity and lighter taste of food. The nature healing take place better at home than in hospital within the family members. If the disease require isolation or quarantine, no visitor are allowed to stay close to the patient to prevent the spread of the disease.

CHAPTER 3

MONITORING THE HEALTH CONDITION

3.1 BLOOD PRESSURE

High blood pressure in human body will be accompanied by stresses, sedentary bloated, increase of cardiovascular disease, heart attack, kidney failure, stroke or even death. On the other end, low blood pressure symptoms are weak, tired, dizzy faint and coma. The blood pressure is measured by the systolic and diastolic in mm Hg. The systolic is the blood pressure during heart contract while diastolic refers to the blood pressure during normal condition. The systolic/diastolic blood pressure range for reference is given in **Table 1**.

Table 1: Blood pressure in mm Hg

Blood pressure (systolic/diastolic) mm Hg	Stanford Cardiologist classification
210/120 -240/130	Stage 4 Severe high blood pressure
180/110	Stage 3 Severe high blood pressure
160/100	Stage 2 Moderate high blood pressure
140/90	Stage 1 Mild high blood pressure
130/85	High normal
120/80	Normal blood pressure
110/75	Low normal
90/60	Borderline low
60/40	Too low blood pressure
50/33	Danger blood pressure

Diastolic blood pressure of more than 140 mm Hg is important CVD risk factor for people older than 50 years (JNC-7, 2003). The JNC-7 found that every increment of 20/10 mm Hg starting from blood pressure of 115/75 mm Hg double the CVD risk. According to WHO, hypertension affected a billion individuals contribute to the death of approximately 7.1 million. Antihypertensive drug prescribed to the patients in combination of healthy lifestyle able to control hypertension.

Blood pressure is moderated by simple steps of quit smoking habit, reduce weight through regular exercise, consumed food with low salt, low protein, reduced caffeine intake, mild sedentary and have enough sleep and rest.

3.2 GLUCOSE LEVEL

It is very important to have regular glucose check for healthy body condition as the excessive glucose in blood plasma show the imbalance in the metabolic system. The excess glucose is due to the failure of pancreas to produce insulin. The patient is considered as insulin dependence diabetes mellitus or Diabetes Mellitus Type 1 if the patient require insulin dose to control the blood sugar. Type 1 mostly affected younger groups.

Diabetes Mellitus Type 2 occurs due to lack of insulin secreted by the pancreas which is drug base dependence is affected almost 90-95% of all diabetes patients. The blood sugar of more than or equal to 11.1 mmol/L is considered as Diabetes Mellitus Type 2 taken by after 2 hours oral glucose tolerance test (according to IDF, 2005). **Table 2** shows the pre-meal glucose for monitoring the glucose level from CareSens™ logbook using i-sen e-Checker test strip.

Table 2: Pre-meal blood glucose

Blood level	Range of blood glucose
1.1-3.9	Low blood glucose
4.0-6.0	Optimal
6.1-8.0	Ideal
8.1-10.0	Sub-optimal
10.1-33.3	High blood glucose

Lower blood sugar is achievable through eating the lower glycemic carbohydrates, consume whole grains, fruits, vegetables, protein and essential fatty acids containing omega 3. Practice regular exercises to ensure healthy weight loss for preventing the obesity. Say no to trans-fats or reduce the saturated fats intake.

3.3 BODY MASS INDEX

Consider your body is the largest asset you own no matter who you are, so take care of your health by monitoring the condition and health status. The healthy body weight can be measured by Body Mass Index (BMI). The BMI counts body fat based on the weight and height. BMI value is categorized into specific health conditions shown in **Table 3**.

The waist circumference reflects possible health risk of overweight and obesity. Higher risk is expected with waist size of greater than 32 inches for women and greater than 40 inches for men. The health risk associated to obesity are high blood pressure, high LDL cholesterol, low HDL cholesterol, high triglycerides, high blood sugar, family history of premature heart disease, physical inactivity and cigarette smoking.

Table 3: BMI Categories (NIH, 2015)

Relative health condition	BMI
Underweight	<18.5
Normal weight	18.5-24.9
Overweight	25.0-29.9
Obesity	≥ 30

BMI in the range of 20-25 is considered as ideal and associated with low risk of disease. The risk of disease is intensified as BMI increases with more chances of developing disease are exposed to men (Giampapa et al., 2004).

3.4 TONGUE DISCOLORATION

The tongue shows some clue on the internal problem inside your body. That why the doctor normally observed your tongue before observe other indicator. Anti-aging expert and Chinese medicine, Dr. Maoshing Ni says that the tongue is one of the important diagnostic areas. The tongue is divided into 5 areas, the front tip, behind the tip, right, left and center. Each corresponds to specific organs and body element. The tip part represents the heart related to fire element. The left and right of the tongue refer to the liver and gall bladder which carry the wood element. Behind the tip is the lung reflection with indicate the metal element. Center part is for the spleen and stomach area represent by earth element. Back of the tongue is the kidney, bladder and intestines reflection areas which governed by the water element.

The discoloration or odd appearances on tongue surface reflex illnesses. Healthy tongue is light to medium pink. The body illness or conditions related to the tongue discoloration is described in **Table 4**. The tongue map in **Figure 2** indicates the taste, element and representative internal organs areas on the tongue surface.

Table 4: Tongue discoloration and associated illness or body conditions

Color of Tongue or Appearance	Illness or Body Conditions
Scarlet or purple	Inflammation, infection or hyperactivity form raising heat
Bright red	Inflammation from excess heat generated from spicy food, smoking or drinking or even stress
Pale tongue	Body is in weak condition, cold, low energy or anemia
Coated tongue	Mucus coated on tongue surface due to slow digestion and weak digestion, or due to dehydration or fungal infection

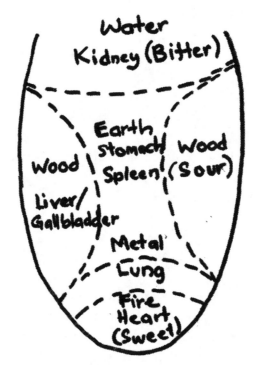

Figure 2 The tongue map

CHAPTER 4

COSMETIC AND SKINCARE

4.1 HARMFUL ADDITIVES

Most of the cosmetic and skincare products are loaded with chemicals compounds for different reason some for colorants, other for stabilizer or to enhance shelf life. The effect of these chemical may cause dizziness, fatigue and muscle damage.

Many chemicals found in the consumer products considered as harmful ingredients are widely used for numerous functions which may interrupts internal organs or create health problems.

The following compounds are part of the consumer product's ingredient:

1. Petrolatum added in lip balms has photosensitivity effect and interfere the body's moisturizer preventing the skin surface from breathing.
2. Polysorbate is used as emulsifier can cause health problem such as drowsiness, nausea, headaches, vomit and irritation, if ingested, inhaled or absorbed through the skin.
3. Propylene glycol permeates skin as moisture carrier used in household products has the negative effect of skin as this ingredient is a strong irritant or over dosage application caused liver and kidney damage. The propylene glycol is used as solvent or surfactant in adhesives, coolants, varnishes, rubber cleaners and shampoo.
4. Methyl, propyl, butyl and ethyl paraben added for extending the shelf life or microorganisms control in products are toxic compounds. The chemicals may cause allergic and skin rashes. Parabens disrupt endocrine system in human body by changing the hormone balance. The imbalance hormone in women which resulted in excessive estrogen formation will change the physical appearance such due to weight gain, or developed stress and affect emotional stability.
5. Imidazolidinyl urea and diazolindinyl urea are used as preservatives which may cause dermatitis due to its skin irritant and allergens effect.

6. pvp/va copolymer is the ingredient found in the hair spray or cosmetic may deposit in the lungs system.
7. Carbomer 934, 940, 941, 960 and 961 added to the cosmetic for thicken the products may cause eye irritation.
8. Sodium lauryl sulfate, sodium laureth sulfate, ammonium lauryl sulfate commonly added to shampoo, soap and facial cleanser as foaming agent. The same materials are used in car wash and detergent products. The usage of products containing SLS can cause eye irritation, skin rashes, hair loss, scalp scurf, allergic reaction, neurotoxicity, endocrine disruption, biochemical changes, mutation and cancer.
9. Stearalkonium chloride found in hair conditioners and creams can cause allergic reactions.
10. Synthetic colors such as Blue 1, Green 3, Yellow 5, 6 and Red 33 are carcinogenic that may developed cancer when ingested or absorbed onto skins.
11. Synthetic fragrances may cause headaches, dizziness, rash, hyperpigmentation, coughing, skin irritation, cancer, vomiting, nerve damage and birth defect.
12. TEA-lauryl sulfate used in shampoo form synthetic detergents,
13. Triethanolamine is pH adjuster, thickener and foam booster can causes allergic reaction to the eye, hair or skin due to toxic property. Diethanolamine (DEA) in shampoo may contribute to potent carcinogen of NDEA when contaminated with nitrites. DEA also block the absorption of choline nutrient which retard brain development.
14. Formaldehyde used as preservative in shampoo is toxic and irritant to the skin.
15. Alpha-hydroxyl acids used as anti-aging ingredient able to remove skin outer layer for delicate and young appearance but leave premature skin exposed to the chemical which accelerate the aging effect.
16. Mineral oil is used for cutting fluid and lubricants. The oils coated the skin and clog the pores inhibit natural oil and caused skin dehydration.
17. Collagen has large molecules that coated the skin surface and cause skin dehydration due to inhibition of natural oil.
18. Alkyl-phenol ethioxylades is additive in shampoo and the frequent used can lower sperm count.
19. MSG may also be added in the shampoo but using different names such as amino acid, glutamic acid or glutamates. The use of MSG may cause headaches, dizziness, nausea, weakness and numbness.

All of these chemicals were added as part of ingredients in shampoo, lip balm, facial cleanser and face cream for different purposes as preservative, anti-caking, colorant, foaming agent, filler or for specific advantages as anti-aging and smooth coverage.

4.2 CREATE YOUR OWN COSMETIC

The safest way for long term benefit is to utilize the natural based cosmetic for healthy skin from kitchen ingredients.

The preparation of kitchen cosmetic requires the essential oils, dilution oils, beeswax, lanolin, honey, fruits, milk, yogurt, cereals and container (amber bottles). Suitable essential oils for oily skin may include Calendula, Geranium, Horsetail, Sage and Yarrow. In case of dry or sensitive skin, borage, cornflower, houseleek, Lady's Mantle, Marsh Mallow, Sorrel and Sweet Violet can be used as a blend in skin care products. Given here few simple ingredients for blending the face toner, face cream, masks, skin purifier, water bath, massage oil and body scrub.

1. Toner: 25 drops essential oil according to your skin type, 100 ml distilled water or rose water. Pour water in the amber bottle and add in essential oil continue by shaking well for 2-3 minutes.
2. Face cream:4-6 drops of essential oil, 7 gm beeswax, 60 ml sweet almond and 30 ml distilled water or rose water. Heat beeswax and sweet almond oil in a bowl stir over a pan of boiling water until melts, remove the bowl and continuously stirring the mixture. Add essential oil and let the blend cool to ambient temperature while continue stirring. Store the cream in amber bottle.
3. Clay mask: 1 drop essential oil, 1 tsp kaolin or fuller earth and 5 ml of rose water or distilled water. Blend the kaolin with water in a small bowl, add in the essential oil and mix well.
4. Fruit mask: 1 drop of essential oil, 1 tsp of ripe fruit or can used yogurt. Mash the fruit and sieve into a small bowl, add essential oil and mix well the selected ingredient.
5. Massage oil: Few drops of selected essential oils in carrier oil of almond oil, coconut oil, olive oil.
6. Toning mask: Blend until smooth half of avocado fleshes and few green grapes, add in honey, lemon, lime, whole egg, and finally put in the baking soda and mayonnaise. The mask will tones and refresh the tired skin on the face.
7. Skin purifier: Put few saffron filaments in a cup of hot milk for 15 minutes for skin vitality and purity. Use the milk to moist the face and let it dry on skin before wash off.
8. Aromatic water bath: Add in the fragrance flowers in bathtub consist of rose, jasmine, ylang-ylang, natural salt and few drops of essential oils according to your suitability. Sit in the bath tub while experience the aromatic smell around you.
9. Body scrub: Use a cup of gluttonous rice powder and soak into water for 72 hours in tamarind juice and the scrub is ready to use for a smooth skin.

10. Make-up removal: Use milk or plain yogurt to remove make-up from your face. Use the wetted cotton ball with the blend of olive oil, castor oil and canola oil to remove make-up on delicate areas around the eyes.
11. Blackhead: Use honey oatmeal and egg white to cleanse and remove the blackhead.
12. Astringents: Use cucumber juice or mashed pulps or diluted lemon as astringent
13. Cleansing grain: Almond powder, oat and orange peel for face scrub.
14. Facelift: Apply honey on face and covered with fruit blend consist of strawberry, grape, orange and apple. Let dry before rinse with cold water.
15. Lotion: Blend peach to get the juice and mix with fresh cream and cool in refrigerator before use.
16. Reducing pores: Use buttermilk with salt or almond paste on face until dry and cleanse with warm water before rinse with witch hazel or apple cider vinegar solution.

Chapter 5

Nutrients for Health Maintenance

5.1 Recommended Daily Allowance

According to Recommended Daily Allowance (RDA) for requirement of human nutrition, the intake of vitamin and minerals for healthy adult should come with complete dosage listed in **Table 5**. In reality, the complete diet is rare but achievable by those who can afford to pay. The RDA is prepared as guidances to the public people. Even though complete nutrient were available in capsule or pill but it is not advisable to take the complete nutrient through this way. The original source of organic nutrient will provide a healthier choice. There is a fact that the calcium consume in a pill is not delivered to the appropriate target organ but was misunderstood by the body system by sending to the wrong target points, the arteries, causing hardening of the artery wall and finally block the passage of blood flow. As a result the consumption of calcium pill has caused to the heart attack problem.

Table 5: RDA Vitamin and minerals for adults

Vitamin and minerals	RDA in mg	Purposes
B1	1.9	Metabolic reactions
B2	1.8	Energy metabolism coenzyme
Niacin	20	Energy metabolism coenzyme
B6	2	Amino acid metabolism
Panthothenic acid	5-10	Energy metabolism
Folacin	0.40	Nucleic and amino acid metabolism coenzyme
B12	0.003	Nucleic acid coenzyme
Biotin	0.15-0.30	Fat synthesis, amino acid metabolism and glycogen formation

Choline	500-900	Phospholipids constituents, precursor or neuro-transmitter acetylcholine
C	45	Cartilage bone and dentine maintenance, collagen synthesis
A	1	Visual pigment and epithelial tissues maintenance
D	0.01	For bone and mineralization; calcium absorption
E	15	Antioxidant and prevent cellular damage
K	0.03	Blood clotting
Calcium	800	Bone and tooth formation; blood clotting; nerve impulse transmission
Phosphorus	800	Bone and tooth formation; acid base balance
Chlorine	2000	Acid-base balance; body water balance; nerve function
Sodium	2500	Formation of gastric juice; acid-base balance
Magnesium	350	Acid-base balance; body water balance; nerve function
Iron	10	Activation of enzymes in protein synthesis
Flourine	2	Constituent of hemoglobin and enzymes for energy metabolism
Zinc	15	
Iodine	0.14	Bone structure maintenance
Water	1.5 L	Constituent of enzymes involve in digestion Constituent of thyroid hormones Metabolic reaction and transport of nutrient; body regulator

5.2 FOOD FOR THOUGHT

One of the important fact is that taking too much of sugar tend to degrade the mental ability. A study by University of California, Los Angeles found that high dose of processed fructose (such as corn syrup in many soft drink, processed food and condiment) can damage memory and learning ability which is dissimilar to the natural fructose from fruit. Luckily the counter effect was shown by taking the docosahexaenoic acid (DHA). DHA help brain cell transmit signals to one another.

The important brain chemicals include acetylcholine, GABA, serotonin, dopamine, endorphins, tyramine, taurine, prostaglandins, purinenecleosides, neropinephrine and certain peptides.

The peanut contains monounsaturated fat, folate, magnesium, potassium, saponin and resveratrol and phytosterols which can lower the blood cholesterol, improve cognitive ability, reduce cancer and heart disease.

Asparagus is known as brain tonic, contain fructo-oligosaccharides (FOS) that help regulate the cholesterol levels. Asparagus also contain folate and vitamin E.

The brain power herbs to improve mind energy can be used in the combination of peppermint, Siberian ginseng, skull cap, wood betony, gotu-kola and kelp prepared as tea.

5.3 Brain Damaging Habits and How to Optimize Brain Functionality

Don't skip the breakfast in early day since we have overnight rest without food. This will lower the blood sugar as in the morning from 7-9 am absorption of nutrients in the small intestine is expected. Overeating causes hardening of brain arteries and decrease mental power. High sugar consumption will interrupt the absorption of protein and nutrients and interfere with brain development.

Prevent the exposure to air pollution, which reduce the supply of oxygen to the brain and affected to decrease in agility or mental efficiency. The harmful smoke from cigarette may cause brain shrinkage and Alzheimer disease.

Sleeping habits will determine healthy brain, either lacks of sleep or overslept can reduced the brain functionality. The average of 8 hours for adult is enough for rejuvenation process and regeneration of cell. Regular sleep time and pattern is advisable for good concentration and mental acuteness.

Finally the brain is fuel by special exercise to stimulate the mental challenge for regeneration and active brain cell functionality. The exercise can be in the form of solution to a new games, or puzzle, life survival and can trigger mental creativity expansion of new horizon and spur excitement to the neuron cell.

The liver damage is affected by the same reasons as mentioned before and including the consumption of too much food additives, overcook or raw food.

Human body has time-based rhythm or functional regulator cycle. This unique cycle has specific time frame for performing regular task automatically except if it encounter disturbance elements. Up to certain level our body can adjusted accordingly such as night shift work scheduled but it can affect to health for long term task where the antibody system might be reduced. The specific times for performing regular body maintenance are:

1. 1-3 am detoxification process in the gall ideally done in deep sleep
2. 3-5 am detoxification in the lung sign by the severe cough for the sufferer
3. 5-7 am detoxification in the colon

4. 7-9 am time for breakfast as nutrients absorption by small intestine is taking place and to stay fit early breakfast is advisable or those who is sick
5. 9-11 pm detoxification from antibody system (lymph node), at this time the best use for relaxing or listening to music
6. 11pm-1am detoxification of the liver which ideally done in a deep sleep state

You can improve the antibody of your body by specific massage on the feet for upper body part and lower part at the right and left side of your sole. To improve the vitality and activate all nerve system and blood vessel in the upper part of body, massage upward from the fingertip to the shoulder. Perform the same massage to the left hand with the right hand. Next step, to increase antibody of higher body part, massage the back of the leg until back of the thigh in upward movement using both hands. The massage is best practiced during early morning or afternoon where the nerve and muscle is in soft condition.

For Muslim, the ablution steps perform before proceed to the prayer has many beneficial effects to improve the blood circulation. One of the important steps is cleaning the face. In this face cleansing, a nerve point at the top left and side of the forehead is pressed by both thumb in toward the hair line to rejuvenate the skin. The final steps of washing the feet promote body's immune system through massaging the lower and upper parts of antibody points. A western massage discover on distress by gentle pinch on the eyebrow using both hand for left and right eyebrows.

Experiencing depression is not an easy moment for all, life expectation seems restricted and distorted during depression attack and mental preoccupied will distract reality. Physical behavior may changes into more aggressive and rational thinking easily fades by chronicle mind.

Numerous sources of stresses relieved are available. I have discovered few effective stresses relieves from traditional methods or moderns activities that are able to remove stress effect given in preceding Section 6.2.

Continues effort of any proven method will bear fruitful effect which can transform your image plus other advantages of freedom from major disease which involve financial saving on medicines cost.

The day when you review all incidents you had run through, then you will realize how good you have treated your own body by giving the best thing in life nothing more nothing less that you will wish in life rather than healthy body, peaceful mind and lean posture.

5.4 ELEMENTS IN OUR BODY

Human bodies consist of mainly four elements, namely earth, water, fire and metal. All elements blend in a body may influence the character of personal behavior and values.

Varieties in human personal traits bring richness to this world. The Malays practitioner believes that the present of air trap in between the vessel and nerve may disturbed the mental stability where in most of the cases affected to the mother after childbirth especially with the presence of air in the empty uterus. I have been thought by a friend for a clue of excess air in our body simply by looking at palm skin color. The pale white spot on the palm shows trap air inside our body and create problem which can make you suffers such as headache.

Stressful condition develop in one body is indicated by the intense nerve at the base of the thumb. The problem is counter by gentle massage from the base of index finger to the base of the thumb on the patient's palm which will soften the intense nerve. Where does the air come from? The organic food and beverages that we ate are releasing few gases and trap in our digestion system has move into the specific muscle and nerves.

A claim from the infra-red (IR) slimming suit designer that the IR can remove air and cholesterol in our body was still ambiguous as Australian government has banned for the usage of IR machine for sunbathing due to the cancer risk. The healthy ways to remove the air is by Shiatsu massages which activate the acupuncture points.

Another method to relieve the stress using Emotional freedom technique (EFT) introduced by Dr Mercola which can also reduce obesity. (http://eft.mercola.com). The method activates acupressure point at the energy meridians to treat emotional health by fingertip tapping. The user of EFT will have the advantage of negative energy removal, reduced food craving, reduce or eliminate pain as well as for implement the positive goal.

Other essential element for healthy mind and body is water. We need to consume enough clean water. Most tap water contains chlorine residual originated from chlorine dosage as disinfectant in water treatment plant. The chorine residual can react with carbon groups and forming carbon tetrachloride (CCl_4) which is carcinogenic and can cause cancer. The maximum CCl_4 is control at 3 microgram per liter according to WHO standard. Trihalomethanes (THMs) also formed from the reaction of chlorine with decay organic material can adversely effects the liver, kidney, central nerve system and cause cancer. Water quality in the water reservoir is contaminated by the residues from agricultural activity, industrialization and urbanization. Aluminum residue in the tap water can caused dementia, kidney failure and stroke.

The presence of heavy metals in the water namely lead, mercury and cadmium may cause health effect to the human body. Lead can impair cognitive level and neurological behavior at 0.05 mg/L. Cadmium can disrupt brain function and effect skin, causing gastric, diarrhea, red eye, headache, difficult breathing, loss of tooth, amnesia, memory loss, cancers and kidney disease at low level of 0.005 mg/L. The accumulation of mercury at the maximum limit of 0.001 mg/L in water can disrupt body functions and lead to death. The tap water must be filtered for potable water usage. A good water filtration system should include the carbon filter, colloidal filter and disinfection method.

Water therapy was used to release various kinds of diseases by drinking up to four glass of water regularly in the early morning according to Dr Rajeev Sharma, an eminent consultant in homeopathy, yoga, naturopathy and alternative medicine in India. Water will liquidize the body and remove the accumulated toxin. Water can help in cognitive ability as water molecule can transfer memory.

Water is very dynamic molecules, which can change in states and being a universal solvent for many reactions. Water is used in Malays traditional medicine as medium to heal and purify the soul from any negative energy or spirit. Water is magnetize to promote the plant growth or for healing purpose.

Fresh source of oxygen is very important in sustaining healthy life. Oxygen absorb during respiration is the elixir element represent the energy for the soul. In certain circumstances we may face deficient supplement of oxygen. Source of oxygen deficient in human body is summarized in **Figure 3** which contributed from different stressor leading to the health problem.

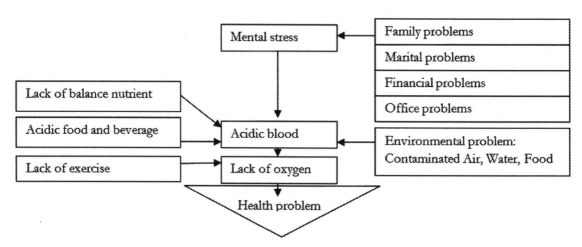

Figure 3: Sources of oxygen deficient

The stressor that causes acidic blood includes lack of balance nutrients, acidic food and beverage, personal problems that contribute to mental stress and environment problems. Health problem easily affected individuals with lack of exercise and at the same time have acidic blood condition.

A quote about life is "Consider the challenge in your life like the dew dance on the leaves" every single thing happen to you is happening with purpose for something good in future. All problems we face has it time period, consider it temporary. Then you don't have to worry just because you have a problem, wait for it time period to end.

Chapter 6

Health Inhibitors

There are so many factors that have some kind of influence to the health. Obviously, financial problem related to owning debts, from the overspending or over budget behavior. Financial planning will help controlling the spending by lives under your means. Utilize money wisely and do spending if you think you can afford to pay for your purchasing. If you spend lavishly you are making other people rich, the seller who received your money! Differentiate between the need and the wishes lists of item or material to help you on prioritized the spending. The need is your vital material to help you continue your lives, but the wishes only give extra comfort by having the material or asset. If you have piles of debts you kept on worrying on how to settle all the debts. Mind energy is disturbed by thinking negative thought so as your health affected by weaken the body's energy to perform work efficiently.

Harmonized relationship with family, friends and colleagues promote good health especially for young people. Abuse in any role will give adverse health effect which finally distorted the life perspective and metal clarity which lead to mental disorder. Life is taking toll when there is a gap in understanding the one's own responsibility toward other. The crime rate has dramatically increases such as pick pocketing, robbery and cheating as life perception change into monetary and material focus. When the material wishes list is limitless but lack of purchasing power has force third option, rob as a choice rather than owned with dignity. There must be paradigm shift of mind focus from materials into spiritual believes. Life must be faced with reality that all matter serves it purposes well without unnecessary materials. Clear perception and moderation in dealing with the essential and luxury wishes list should be inculcated to the young generation.

The recent trends in skin beauty become priority for many ladies and men. Actually we have been created with all the complete beauty, but most of us think if we can use collagen to make skin smoother, using skin whitening to look fairer but it only can happen with the sacrifice of food sources, plant and animal cells just to satisfy the wealthy groups as they afford to pay is not justifiable. Excessive uses of the food products as cosmetic ingredients will cause the rise on food price and bring difficult life for the poorer.

6.1 STRESS DEVELOPMENT

At work there are a lot of factors that contribute to stress, unexpected reaction from a given load or situation to a man (Dr David B Posen-lifestyle counselor and psychotherapist). Stress exists in form of challenge, threat, or any changes which require the individual adaptation. Stress may give a positive, 'eustress', or a negative, 'distress' effect toward personal outcome. The stress may bring a new discovery due to the exertion of mental power to solve specific problem. In history, communication system was designed by Alexander G Bell in his attempt to help his fiancé loss of hearing (Stephen C Phillips). There are three categories of stress factor (Desai, 1999):

1. Physiological
2. Psychological
3. Environmental

The physiological factors are inherited genetic and congenital factors, bad life experience, shifted or disturbed normal biological rhythm causing fatigue, muscular pain. Meanwhile the psychological factors include individual perception, emotion, situation, sensation, decision, memory, motivation, cognition and appraisals. Environmental factors are associated to the ambient environment, physical event, social event, and biotic events. The latter factors also contributed by the psychological and physiological sub-system.

During stress our body produce adrenaline into blood vessel and body adapted to the stress by accelerate of heart rate and the increase of blood pressure to pump into the brain and muscle this will cause more sugar, fat and cholesterol in blood to provide more energy. Continuing the stress situation will contribute to the disease of heart attack and stroke. Extra fatty acid found in blood will be converted into fat and cholesterol which covered the blood vessel thus increase the heart attack and stroke (HEA, 1996, Stress and heart disease). Stress effect may also contribute to the insomnia, diabetes, gastric, ulcer, infection and asthma. Prozac is one of the stress relieve drug that change the brain chemical by enhance the serotonin level. Stress actually do damage DNA by shortened the telomeres, the protective binder in the DNA cell strand. About 30 percent of the workers are reported to have extreme stress levels. According to American Psychological Association, two-third of the Americans quoted that job as a main source of stress in their lives.

Stress management is important knowledge for all workers to equip themselves with the methods and techniques to face the stressful conditions.

6.2 Stress Relieves Methods

There are five types of coping strategies in dealing with developed stress, cognitive, behavioral, social, avoidance and religious/spiritual approach. Cognitive approach is initiated by analyzing the problem for the possible course of action and select effective plan after evaluating the efficacy. Other cognitive solution is derived by self-talk to stimulate formulation and implementation of coping strategies and provides corrective feedback. The third method is by reappraisal the impact of stressful event by different meaning or interpretation. Behavioral approach involves the personal response toward the stress by finding the event details, take immediate action or inhibiting action or turning to others. The latter response was also known as social approach whereby the social support provides solution to the problem.

Avoidance strategy is used in the condition of threatening stressor or scarce resources. Personal in stressful condition try to avoid the tension through taking drugs, excessive eating or drinking or smoking. The last strategy, religious/spiritual believes is one of the useful approach as in religious practice especially during prayer, the alpha state is achieved if the person has strong believes of their fate have been written from the beginning of the life journey.

Whatever interferences faces during one's life journey has nothing to do with back luck or negative karma, the problem happen for goodness benefit in stored for you in the future life journey. The reason of unpleasant thing happens to you today because it will be rewarded later when you are in emergency situation. Through religion, the faith of universe is unveiled for those who open their mind to explore all the factual of life.

Simple steps to immediately relieve stress may include the following techniques:

1. Communicate with the trusted personnel who can hear your problem and guide for solution. A stressful condition will be released simply by sharing with friend or family member. It is practically normal to seek a shoulder to cry on for listening to your stressful problems.
2. Try to find peaceful environment where lot of positive charges are available to purify the negative energy in your minds such as close to waterfall and seashores. Enjoy the sound of water fountain or wave's motion can also soothe your mind.
3. Express the negative condition or problem by writing or a sketch on a piece of paper and put the paper in an envelope and throw away the enveloped on moving water like sea or river.

4. Release the stress by following the tough sport like climbing, swimming or jungle trekking where you can use the large amount of energy on the sport.

5. Have enough sleep every night from 8 to 7 hours for men and women. Since during the sleep period, the body's cells repairs the damaging effect during the daylight and recharge for the next day process. During the sleep subconscious mind is still functioning for your success of what you have affirmed to your mind before bedtime. The mind itself is the source of energy. If you know how to capitalize your own energy it will work for you well.

6. Laughter is the best medicine. Gelotheraphy will increase the oxygen to your blood. It can promote the alertness and relaxation which improve the brain function. Laughter also improves the immune system effectiveness, reduce anxiety and tension.

7. Detoxify your liver using citrus blend with olives oil and ginger. It is useful to flush out the accumulated toxin in liver. It will make your face become reddish with glows since more blood flow to face after purification in your liver.

8. Buy yourself a gift before you provide gift to others. Appreciate your own achievement even nobody bother to gift you any token. A way to appreciate your values, your presence and your effort to please yourself is a way of healing by something that you like or eyes for long times.

9. Empower yourself, by attractive and be attentive to people around you, advised from Georgette Mosbacher, one of the successful business women to turn moment into lifetimes. It will be great personal properties for your futures. Change your outlook to a better state as far you can.

10. Use the traditional massage such as Guasa, Shiatsu or reflexology and use acupuncture points to heal stress and diseases rather than drug healing. These methods can reduce the amount of synthetic chemical consumption which may have long term side effect shown up at the older age.

11. If the stress affected hair loss, you can take supplement of vitamins A, C, E with biotins to promote and strengthening the hair growth.

12. Depression in women due to pre-menstrual symptoms (PMS) is advised to take vitamins B and E, magnesium, zinc and amino acid tyrosine, L-phenylalanine and L-glutamine. PMS depression is cause by estrogen and progesterone imbalance in the endocrine system.

13. Chiropractic practice can help realign the spine system problem where the spinal nerves are connected to the internal organ. Any fracture or slipped disc will badly affected your emotion as well as your comfortability.

14. Use aromatherapy of your choices to revive and uplift your spirit.

15. Depression essential oils: Basil, bergamot, frankincense, geranium, jasmine, lavender, neroli, patchouli, rose and ylang-ylang. Use few drops of the essential oil for massage in almond oil or used a burner to vaporize the oil in your room.
16. Stress essential oils: Basil, lavender, mandarin, marjoram, neroli, orange, petit grain, clary sage and ylang-ylang. Drink tea made of melissa, orange and mint
17. Use anti-stress diet in your food intake.

    a. Reduce the excessive salt in food which is associated with high blood pressure and tendency for water retention.
    b. Take enough vitamin C and B from fruit and vegetables sources to protect your capillary, for protein and fat metabolism as well as produce energy.
    c. Have enough calcium and potassium for bone and muscle from milk, banana, cabbage, grape, apples, corn, lemon, lettuce, water melon, pineapples, plum, pear, orange, peach, cherries, cauliflower and potatoes.
    d. Consume enough plain water to provide for body flushing and regulate healthy waste removal.
    e. Reduce the caffeine intake from tea and coffee and other stimulant like alcohol and nicotine.
    f. Take smaller amount of meal by having more frequent meal for proper digestion.

18. Create a hobby that gives pleasure to you. Living with animal like cat or fish can provide calming effect. The animal will help you in certain way and make healing process faster.
19. Socializing create happiness thorough sharing the story or gathering with family members or friends for celebrating specific functions.
20. Take a holiday break to the remote areas like island, rainforest, beaches and lakes. Visit a new places opened yourself to new experience, new people and new cultures.
21. Enrich yourself with new knowledge, new skill or new languages. Learn to do new thing like crafting, drawing, painting and sewing.
22. Uplift your spiritual believes and thought by prayers or deep meditation. Induce more alpha state in your mind for calming and clear minds.
23. Use materials or object that can improve your environment, change or rearrange the layout, color and shape.

CHAPTER 7

TIP TO STAY AWAY FROM CHRONIC DISEASES

This section is presented to give some simple tips, steps, or way to remove or to protect from world most chronic disease and promote good health. A vital asset for all of us is our own unique body. Take care yourselves before you take care others.

7.1 BALANCING VITAL COMPONENTS

All of the following food components are consumed in predefined balance amount to carry specific body functions. Percentage of consumption may vary as per individual need according to gender and body structure. Follow the recommended food pyramid and choose food according to their recorded glycemic index (GI).

1. Water is part of body component, every day you liquid intake must be from 1.5 to 2 Liters (RDA requirement) based on individual mass weight. Alkaline water is good for our stomach as it will prevent body infections from various diseases. Magnetized water can characterize body shape. Use north poles to stay in slim shape or south poles for more oval shape.
2. The intake of caffeinated water requires double the intake of plain water. Water also can hold memory, so if you are in learning process, drink enough water as fluid can accelerate learning process. Water remove as sweat can remove toxin it good for your body. Most of the antioxidants are water soluble which help to transfer the bio-molecule into internal organ for health benefit.
3. Take sugars with fibers to eliminate the sugars been deposit as fat. The fibers will help prevent the formation of diabetic condition. Natural sugar contains nutrient compared

to processes sugars or white sugar. The white sugar has been acidified to remove natural color. Excessive sugar intake may lead to obesity.

4. Protein has long molecules which make digestion become difficult. The digestion of red meat will produce uric acid causing arthritis due to the deposit of the acid in the tendon muscles. The intake of protein should be limited to appropriate dosage.

5. The cholesterol content in food sources are given in **Table 6**. Recommended daily cholesterol consumption should be no more than 300 mg (American Heart Association).

Table 6: Cholesterol content in variety of multi food sources (MSD)

Type of food	Quantity (g)	Cholesterol (mg)
Meat:		
Lamb (liver)	100	323
Mutton (lean)	100	70
Beef (lean)	100	65
Chicken (breast)	100	39
Sausage (Chinese)	100	150
Seafood:		
Clam	100	65
Squid	100	48
Lobster	100	85
Crab	100	100
Prawn	100	154
Pomfret	100	80
Dairy products:		
Cream	100	140
Cheese	100	100
Butter	100	260
Ice cream	100	45
Milk	100	13
Oil:		
Vegetable oil	100	0
Animal fat	100	74
Egg:		
Egg yolk	1 piece	266
Egg white	1 piece	0
Dug	1 piece	619
Quail yolk	1 piece	74

Vegetables:		
Spinach, cabbage	100	0
Fruits:		
Orange/apple/water melon	100	0
Grain:		
Rice/bread/ macaroni	100	0

Do count the calorie in the food to provide our body energy requirement. The daily calorie need is calculated by basal metabolic rate (BMR). The BMR is the minimum calories the body required to complete body daily function. Calorie expenditure is measured by counting every single pound of body weight which will burns 10 calorie per day and total calories should be factored by individual daily activity and digestion (Gruenemay, 2005). The activity varied according to the nature of individual work as in **Table 7**. The calorie for digestion need is estimated as 10 percent to the final sum of the calorie.

Table 7: Activity factor to account for BMR

Activity	Factor in BMR (%)
Sedentary (sitting and office works)	20
Light activity (infrequent movements)	30
Moderate activity (Lifting and lots of movements)	40
Very active (in sport and athletes)	50

For body weight of 132 Ib (59.87kg) the calories is calculated as:

132 X10 =1320

1320 x 0.2 (sedentary activity) = 264

1320 + 264 = 1584

1584 x 0.1 =158.4

1584 + 158.4 = 1742.4

The minimum calories for 132 Ib body weight after account for activity and digestion will be 1742 calorie. Effective weight loss is achieved by the balance between less calorie food intake and the fat burning activity such as 30 minutes brisk walking or gardening. High caloric fruits are banana (1 medium size) and dates (5 pieces) have 110 and 120 calorie accordingly (Moss Greene, 2015) contain multi vitamins and minerals.

6. Fat can behave as two faces coined, there are good fat and bad fat in the food sources. Good fat can heal disease but bad fat can cause problem. Alpha-linoleic acid and linoleic acid are essential fatty acids (EFAs) from fat and oils. The balance intake of these two acids, known as Omega-3 and Omega 6 (2:1) increase the metabolic reaction, energy level and stamina. The existence of 12 to 15% total calories in form of EFAs can help to burn fats and glucose.

The EFAs benefit includes as follows (Erasmus, 2003):

a. lower cancer risk (Omega 3)
b. decrease infection as antifungal, anti-yeast and anti-microbial properties
c. help to prevent osteoporosis
d. improve sleep
e. ease PMS through GLA and Omega 3
f. improve response to stress by optimize serotonin production. Serotonin plays an important role in regulation of mood, sleep, emesis (vomiting), sexuality and appetite.
g. autoimmune conditions
h. reduces allergic symptom

The bad fats are hydrogenated fat found in shortening, margarine, hydrogenated oil after commercial processing at high temperature which forms trans-fatty acid. The negative effects of trans-fatty acid are elevate cardiovascular disease, increase cancer risk and interfere insulin secretion and prostaglandins production.

7. Consume fruit with antioxidants in the fresh shell. The best fruit loaded with nutrient are avocado, grapefruit, kiwifruit, and berries. I used to detoxify the liver using citrus blend with olive oil. We have abundant variety of fruits from tropic or temperate regions which can provide photochemical like polyphenol compound. The phenolic compounds in green plant help to moderate the diabetic effect, used to treat cancer and many other infections.

7.2 Top 5 Fruits for Antioxidants

Selected top 5 fruits rich in vitamin and minerals as antioxidants to fight free radicals and provide many health benefits to the human body.

Avocado – The super fruit contains 20 vitamins and minerals for the well-being from its raw flesh. The fruit provide all vitamin of A, C, D, E, K, B complex thiamine, riboflavin, niacin, panthothenic acid, biotin, B6, B12 and folate required by human body. The energy of 1 oz. flesh avocado is 50 calories and was included in dietary program by many worlds' nutrition bodies. The fruit has been used in cosmetic products and health meals ingredients.

Grapefruit – Healthiest fruit rich in Vitamin C and help in prevent the free radical damage by reduce inflammatory condition from the asthma, osteoarthritis and rheumatoid, improve cardiovascular health, store and heart attack. The fruit contains lycopene (the red color), carotenoid phytonutrient acts as antitumor that fight free radical and prevent cell damage. The fruit also provides potassium, Vitamin A, folate and Vitamin B5. The energy content in half of medium size grapefruit is 41 calories with low GI.

Blueberry – Highest antioxidant content fruit, where the 100 g of fresh blueberry has 5562 trolox equivalents largely from polyphenolic anthocyanidin compound of chlorogenic acid, tannins, myricetins, quarcetin and kaempferol. The berries also contain flavoids such as β-caroteno, lutein and zea-xanthin which can fight the cancer, aging, degenerative diseases and infections. Chlorogenic compounds help in reducing blood glucose in type 2 diabetes mellitus patients. The fresh berries contain vitamin A, C, E and B complex, niacin, pyridoxine, folate and panthothenic acid. Furthermore, berries provide essential minerals of potassium, manganese, copper, iron and zinc. The energy content in 100 g berries is 57 calories.

Banana – High calorie fruit with 80 calories per 100 g is a good diet with soluble fiber 7% of DRA per 100 g. Rich in vitamin A, C, E, K and B complex of thiamine, riboflavin, pyridoxine, panthothenic acid, Niacin and folate. The banana flesh has essential minerals of calcium, copper, iron, magnesium, phosphorus, selenium and zinc. The flavoid antioxidant in banana is lutein, zea-xantin, β and α-carotine acts as protective against free radicals and play a role in aging and various diseases processes.

Grape – Considered as alkaline fruit which is good for stomach conditioner. The alkaline medium prevents the spread of disease, which normally occur in acidic medium. Most bacteria and virus are active in the acidic medium. Grape is good source of vitamin A, C, K and B complex and minerals. Red grape contain resveratrol, powerful antioxidant for protection of colon and prostate cancer, coronary heart disease, degenerative nerve disease, Alzheimer's disease and viral or fungal infection as well as reduce stroke risk. Antioxidant cathechin also found in the white and green grapes for health protection. The energy provide by 100 g of grape is 69 calories.

Fruit comes in different colors provide different groups of phytochemical compounds as shown in **Figure 4**. The green fruits may contain betacarotine, lutein and xeaxanthin help to prevent cancer. Orange or yellow colors fruit also contain betacarotine may improve the body resistance towards disease infections. The red fruits such as water melon and tomatoes have lycopene which can reduce cardiovascular diseases. The blue colors fruit in plum and blueberry contains anthocyanins able to fight the cardiovascular disease and cancer. White color fruit normally rich in Vitamin C and kalium and contain idoles.

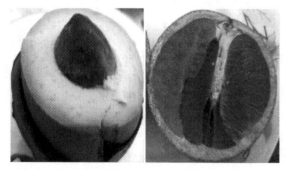

Figure 4 Fruits rich in antioxidants, avocado and grapefruit

7.3 OBESITY EFFECT TO HEALTH AND IMAGES

Obesity or overweight is one of unhealthy lifestyle symptom occur due to few factors such as overeating, lack of physical exercise, inherited genetic and low metabolic function or defective organism mechanism. The social gathering during celebration, parties and formal functions may cause overeating due to abundance food available for consumption. Body responses toward stress, grief, or shock may change eating habit. Obesity is one of the problems in most of developed countries where the advanced technologies are widely used especially for cyber communication using personal computer, hand phone or IT gadgets.

Combination of reduced physical mobility due to modern technology in communication and consumption of fast food can magnify the obesity effects. As all the preservatives, colorants and additives in the fast food or processed food add unnecessary chemicals in human body, which interfere with internal organs function and processes contribute to degenerative diseases in the obese adults. Obesity has shown up to be the global issues as the rate of obesity in 1997 was already 15 to 23% in U.S. and Australia accordingly.

Tendency for obesity also depends on individual body structure known as somatotypes, classify as endomorph, mesomorph and ectomorph. Endomorph figure have round body shape tend to have obesity easily with their short, wide hand and feet skeleton. Mesomorph body has medium figure normally with solid muscle. The third somatotypes, ectomorph body attributed to tall and slim shape rarely face obesity problem.

Obesity changes the appearance of woman figurine into less attractive and appealing. Most women are afraid of being obese especially after married and pregnancy that cause hormone changes for supporting the infant growth. In many cases the body shapes may remain as usual with normal care. Even though obese is well accepted but in reality it is not for the healthy well-being, carrying extra weight tend to suppress the main nerve system and weaken the bones.

In current practice, traditional medicines used for treatment of new mum during the first 40 days after gave birth will ensure the mothers recovery and baby are in healthy conditions. Even the body shape is better compared to virgin posture. It's depends on the emotional state and strong support from family members in taking cares of new members and the mother. The continuous used of special ingredient for maintaining body's shape and health is reflected by shining glory of ageless women. The secret recipe utilize by the older generation has no longer been practiced by the young generation. The younger groups preferred fast and handy health care products available from pharmacy or healthcare outlet.

Obesity increases the risk of metabolic problems such as CVD, diabetes and cancer. Obesity condition is linked to the stress, whereby two out of three adult are overweight or obese with the outcome of significant number of population is being diagnosed with chronic diseases. It is very important to stay in healthy weight and maintain the quality life. Practical suggestions to prevent obesity are:

1. Protein developed muscle and promote body fitness. Eat enough protein in your daily diet.
2. Stress can increase the antioxidant requirement, thus consume fruit fibers with antioxidant from different colors. It provides vitamin, mineral and fibers for good digestion system.
3. Yogurt is good source of vitamin A and Calcium.
4. Drink plain tea or coffee without milk, its good beverage for those who are obese with diabetic.
5. Reduce the intake of fatty pastries, cookies or cakes, as the food contain lots of hydrogenated fat which can increase weight.
6. Hot pepper contains capsaicin which increase metabolic system and thus can help to reduce the weight since the obese people normally have low metabolic rate.

7.4 Techniques on How to Prevent Cancer

Cancer affected one out of 10 populations. The most frequently affected woman is breast cancer while in men is prostate cancer. Nature of cancer development is the same, due to abnormal cell growth which can spread to other organ causing failure of affected organ. Luckily we can reduce the rate of cancer development by many ways, through the food rich in antioxidant content, removal of product with the potential as cancer precursor and have abreast knowledge on the health awareness.

7.4.1 Dairies products

One of the safest ways to prevent cancer formation is through controlling the food intake. The real case of stage four cancer patients, Professor Jane Plant, who was successfully recover from affected cancer through removal of all diaries products in her diet. This includes milk, cheese, and yogurt. Dairies products produce from milk contain higher Insulin Growth Factor, IGF-1 which causes the cells to divide and reproduce. IGF-1 was found at higher level in cow's milk and also found in cow's meat.

7.4.2 Vitamin D

One of the surprising finding by a group of researcher at Mount Sinai Hospital, Toronto Canada proves the relationship between cancer and Vitamin D. Diagnose women with vitamin D deficiency had a 94% increased risk of cancer would spread in their body compared to those who had enough vitamin D. They also found out that the affected patient has 73% risk of dying within the next 10 years. It is easier to get enough Vitamin D from free source, the sun light at 9-12 am or 3-5 pm especially for tropic region.

Vitamin D promotes calcium absorption, essential for nervous and immune systems; and help genes to produce healthy cell growth. Other sources of vitamin D are fish, egg and cereal.

7.4.3 Plastic polymer

The use of plastic packaging in food wrapping can cause cancer due to the release of leached polymer into the food, which produced Bisphenol A (BPA) mainly from polycarbonate plastics as well as other type of plastics products. Plastic molecules are subjected to the scratch and extreme heat in microwave oven will break the polymer bonds which contaminate the food. The BPA as low as 25 part per trillion is enough to show harmful effect. The leach of BPA and phthalate into the food are potential chemicals that disrupt human endocrine systems. The best way to remove these contaminants are by changing all plastic kitchenware and food storage to the glass, ceramic or stainless steel materials.

7.4.4 Health awareness

Healthy habit may prevent you from cancer formation. This includes consumption of fresh foods, fruits and vegetable. Reduce the intake of junk food, preserves food or canned food available in the stores since this kind of food contained MSG, chlorine and hydrogenated fatty foods with the tendency to increase toxin in our body.

Many inherited diseases are associated with the impaired mitochondria function affected aging people like stroke, cancer, diabetes, Aizheimer's disease and heart disease. Body's power plant, mitochondria produce energy together with free radicals which will damage the membrane in mitochondria if the radical is not neutralized by the antioxidant.

Combination of antioxidants intake was found helpful in reducing mitochondria damage are alpha lipoic acid (ALA), acetyl L-carnitine and coenzyme Q10. ALA consumption lowers the oxidative stress in the heart. ALA and acetyl L-carnitine help to improve memory and cognitive performance. The coenzyme Q10 is required to convert fatty acid into energy in the mitochondria cells. The ALA and acetyl L-carnitine tablet form are available in the pharmacy outlet in 150 mg and 400 mg concentration accordingly.

One of popular fruit used to fight cancer is pineapple due the content of bromelain enzyme with antitumor effect superior than chemotherapy drug 5-fluorauracil as quoted in journal Planta Medica based on the animal study. The survival index of tested animal with bromelain is 263% relative to the control.

7.4.5 De-stress activity

Stress tends to accelerate cancer formation and weaken immune systems. Remove stress immediately once you are under stress. Depression tends to reduce mental alertness and delay the body's response toward proper decision making. Understand the source and symptom of the stress help you to manage the stress.

Physical activity like aerobic exercise at least 30 minutes, three times per week to de-stress can refresh the mind and activate energy.

Generate activity that deviate your focus to the stress issues, such as joints the club or become a member in a group, participate in physical fitness, select preferable socializing group like traditional dance, theatre or joint outreach project to help the less fortunate people recovery.

During stress your body release cortisol which used to reduce inflammation during body injury. High cortisol hormone lead to all of the ageing conditions in human body:

1. Loss of memory and cognitive skill
2. High blood pressure
3. Skin degradation
4. Hypogylcemia
5. Metabolic disorder

It is very important to control the stress and counter the stress effect by immediate action bodily and mentally. The meditation can help you see the real situation and find solution to your problem through deeper thought. The solution will appear in your mind for immediate correction. Started with the correct mind then you are already moving toward the practical de-stress.

The changes of your condition after de-stress is associated with the raise in serotonin hormone level. The hormone secreted by pineal gland rise during night time is the control of human biological clock. The big role of the hormone in prevention of DNA damage thus control ageing process. The hormone can be used as appropriate agents for depression relieved. The crystal lamp used at night can promote the serotonin level during deep sleep.

Ayurveda head massages can improve the oxygen circulation and spinal fluid flow through three massages points, the Crown, Brahma Rendra and Karna Marma. The Crown is found about 4 to 5 inches from the top front hair line. The Brahma point is about 2 inches from the crown while the Karna is separated an inch from the second point. The massages points in the head should be rub in clockwise by soft and gentle spiral movement.

The stress removal with the advantages of improve your charismatic power, change negative to positive energy and expand your electromagnetic field is performed by open hand stretching out to the crowd.

Add enough Omega 3 and 6 in your diet as well as food containing tryptophan like banana which is converted into serotonin for release tension and create a happier mood.

CHAPTER 8

SIMPLE STEPS FOR BODY FITNESS AND BEAUTY

There is no short cut secret recipe to the body fitness. The body is aging according to time clock even though some anti-aging product claims that it can prevent all the aging sign, stay young and look young. The best adaptable perception is aging with grace and healthy living. Even for some people they can afford to spend thousand for beautiful products for corrective on the surface appearance but how about their internal organ, liver, kidney and heart which working nonstop to carry specific function which most people forget to look after their very own precious body parts. Remember most of our internal organ has no replacement for any failure or damage. So be kind to your organs and treat them well. But what we can do to give a sense of kind treatment to internal organ? There are numerous techniques available for regulating and simultaneously cleansing the specific organ through food consumption, water flushing and clean air.

Physical fitness is enhanced and developed through the rhythm movement of muscle known in numerous cultures by different name but with almost similar objective and movement. The well-known yoga originated from India, tai chi from Chinese while 'silat' from Malay ethnic. The imitation of tiger or cat movements is observed in many traditional practices for improvement of physical fitness, which received less attention by the young generation. Regular practices of the ancient physical fitness methods hold the secret to enhance three dimensions of life, spiritual, emotional and physical.

8.1 TAI CHI

By practicing tai chi, many positive outcomes can be observed especially for distress and healing purposes. Body's movement is well aligned to tap the environment energy for producing the good effect for regain and replenish. One of the interesting outcomes of Tai chi-chi kung exercise which able to purify and recycle energy through kidney cleansing. The chi kung purification workout is performed in standing position with feet in parallel by shoulder-width apart, place hand on the kidney position and visualize the kidney before shifted the weight toward the left and move waist and arm toward to the right while turning the arm back. Move the arm back to the front. Then turn your waist to face to the left with the arm stretched out. Twist the wrist and float the palm float down while you turned the waist to face forwards. Twist and put back the hand on kidney area. Repeat for the other side with the same steps.

In the second part, while in standing position, places both palm on kidney and shift weight to the left while step forward using right foot 45 degree to the left. Move both arms behind and shifts the weight forward; simultaneously move the arms in front. Bring little finger to point upward and move to the front up close to face level. Finally turn the elbow down slowly to the ground and repeat the previous step for completing the kidney purification.

8.2 ESKAY TECHNIQUE

The stress therapy for athlete or fatigue muscle after heavy duty work was introduced as Eskay technique by provides effective touch program through applied pressure from foot method on specific parts of strain ligaments. The foot pressure is applied to the back, thigh, or leg muscle using either both feet or only one foot of your spouse. The immediate release of the pain can be experienced after repeated pressure given to the affected muscles.

8.3 REFLEXOLOGY

The foot massage can be used for body healing as the nerves on the foot represent various upper part organs. The reflexology map of the relevant organ is useful for giving specific treatment by foot massage through 62 reflexology points. The foot massage introduced in Egypt was popular in China, Europe and United States is one of the safest ways to improve health and longevity. It is good to remember the phrase of the longer you walk the better your health. Practices brisk walk of at least 10,000 steps a day for a healthier body and use pedometer to record the steps while walking.

8.4 REJUVENATION TIPS FOR REVERSE AGING

People with good habits can generally live longer and help them stay young. The good habits are having enough laughs and fun in a day and don't be gloomy. Let bygones be bygones.

Accept the bitter moment in the past with openness and move on with the positive outlook for current and future undertakings. Time wait for no men. Other good habit is early to bed early to rise is healthy and wise practiced. Do something you like, a hobby for earning, or learn something new to stay active even after retirement.

The interest will spur your mind with happiness. It will promote motivation that keeps you young, alert and responsive. Try to prevent consumption of too many pills as it is not good for your body. Stay healthy by regular exercise, quit smoking and eat less fatty food.

Most of aging conditions is contributed by glycation whereby the protein surface is coated by oxidized glucose thus preventing the intended function. The glycation effects may include, memory loss, depression due to disruption of neurotransmitter function, cortisol receptor damage; hormone imbalance, skin sagging or wrinkling, impaired immune functions, causing allergies, impaired gastrointestinal functions and reduced digestion capacity.

The stress condition normally will show up on the palm by the existence of tense nerve in between the thumb and index fingers. The nerve can be found by gentle pressure using reverse thumb in that area. The tense nerves which indicate stress development inside our body can be reduced by massaging the palm in semi-cycle under the index finger to the based on the thumb. Enhance the body immunity by reflexology massage on body's antibiotic points illustrated in **Figure 5** at three location on the foot namely A for the upper part of body, B the stomach and C the chest antibiotic points.

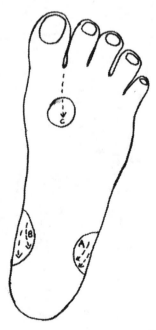

Figure 5: Antibiotic points on upper part of the foot, A, B and C

8.5 HOW TO BOOST FLAWLESS SKIN

The skin is the largest surface that used for protecting the inner body and internal organ. The skin can reflect the internal organs disorder by its colors, skin spot and moles. Even the ancient practitioner can decode complication suffered in the internal organ through the skin surface appearance. Luckily imperfect skin can be corrected through several ways.

Frequent message to the muscle below the breast in downward movement and outward cycles at the back of you hip can improve overall skin vitality, clarity and better body fluidity.

The most practical methods to improve the skin can simply be achieved by reflexology massages. The face treatment by reflexology is done by massaging the foot at several points, number 13, 15, 16, 18, 21 to 25 and 34 from the **Figure 6**. The points reflex the individual organs systems of parathyroid gland, stomach, duodenum, liver, adrenal gland, kidney, ureters, bladder, small intestines and spleen.

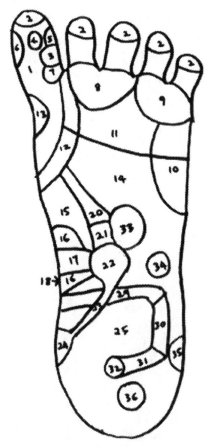

Figure 6 Left foot reflexology points

CHAPTER 9

BEAUTIFUL FIGURE PRACTICES

9.1 FACELIFT

Practice the facelift for toning the weak muscle and sag. The muscle is dropped due to gravity and the weakness of skin elasticity. The counter effect of gravity can be found in the yoga practice in the reverse posture as well as the prostrate position in the Muslims prayer which helps in rejuvenation of the face muscle as well as other body muscles besides relieving stress. Practicing regular reverse position or prostrate help in blood regulation, and minimize the dementia effects at old age.

Facelift can be practiced regularly to strengthen the face muscle (Benz, 1991) which can reduce the fore head wrinkle, eye crow's-feet and laugh lines. The simplified face lift steps are as illustrated in **Figure 7**. Correct facelift can change the shape of face due to fatty muscle along the jaw line into finer shapes for younger appearance.

The massages on face are depicted by the stretch line performed in the direction according to the arrow point. The dotted lines required a localized soft pressure using either middle or index finger without massage. The forehead massage removes the vertical and horizontal lines. The hair lines soft pressure used to rejuvenates the whole face. Similarly the massages on ears promote longevity.

The faces determine your career success, so you can enhance the face attributes by make-up and correct the eyebrows. The color of your face should be appropriate for your occasion and climate. In temperate region the pale face should be highlighted and shaded using suitable foundation after moisturizer application to protect the skin. With the bright sunlight in tropic region, more SFP protection is required and sweat will interfere with the moisturizer or facial creams. Uplift by makeup can help to gives matt or velvet finish which depends on the makeup blend, either oily or water based. I used the water based for my skin, not only because of the oily skin but water can blend well with most of water soluble vitamins like vitamin C.

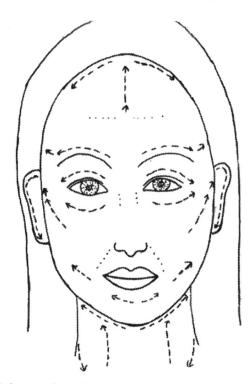

Figure 7: Face-lift to reduce the wrinkle and strengthening face muscles

The soft chin massage upward toward the cheekbone can prevent formation of double layer chin. The soft vibration around the lip can refresh the lip. Light compress on the cheek and cheekbone are able to remove the wrinkle on the cheek and nose areas.

Massage the eye from mid of the nose toward the ears few times with soft hand pressure. The eyes also can be refreshed soon after wake up in early morning by rolling the eyeball in cycle from left to right and, up and down. It is good practice, if the eyes are exposed to morning sunlight for 10 minutes. Always imagine there is a star in between your eyebrow as this will promote your inner shine.

9.2 BREATHING PRACTICE

You need full energy from the oxygen in the inhalation process. Practice full breathes through the nose deeply and slowly for vitality and to remove toxin from our body. Fast and shallow breath will lead to many health problems such as fatigue, sleep disorder, anxiety, and stomach upset. The breathing practice should be exercised twice a day in the morning and afternoon or at night with empty stomach. The alternate breathing between left and right nostril will supply enough oxygen to the brain for creative and analytical thinking, improve personality and balance the emotion. It was believe that if you start your first step in the morning while breathing from right nostril your wishes will come true while the reverse thing will occur if you use the left nostril. Complete the breathing cycle by inhale through each nostril but relieve out the air through the mouth. The deep inhalation of fresh air should be hold for few seconds before exhale for rejuvenation of internal organ especially in the morning while on meditation position. I used to take the break of 8 seconds in between the inhalation cycle.

9.3 TONING MUSCLES

There is an exercise known as sweet lotus worth practiced especially for married women to firm the waistline and toning the buttock muscle. The exercise consists of 8 steps which can be performed in laying position on a thin mat. Bring your ankles in upright posture and hold tightly your leg for 5 seconds. In the next step take a deep breath and lifting up your head to reach the knees and hold for 5 seconds.

The third step promotes rejuvenation started from laying position before sit up for bending to your knees by flatten stomach. After position three, sit back from the bending posture, cross the legs and try to hug your body by pull your face toward left knee then change to right knee. Release the hugging step and straiten your leg, fold your leg as close as possible over the other leg while straighten you hand to hold to reach the toes, inhale slowly and contract your stomach and pelvic floor muscle.

Another exercise to lift the buttock is sitting like the athlete getting ready for marathon then lowers your body to the ground until your thigh touch the stomach, while the other leg is straighten outside lift up your head as far as possible.

The next steps is for stress removal performed by laying in interior position, lift the head and chest as far as possible inhale slowly and let the stomach remain on the floor. The final posture is to tighten your uterus by push up your chin using both hands while in the similar position as in the previous step, simultaneously, grip the heel using the first and second toes of your leg.

Practice the rejuvenation massage for the two point at the back of your waist by putting your both hand hold the waist and used only the thumb to cycle the waist and the massage point below the breast in downward movement using both hand with anticlockwise and clockwise cycle for right and left side simultaneously.

Simple steps to toning and tightening the buttock, thigh, waistline and stomach muscles are illustrated in **Figure 8**. Regular practice will help your body stay in good posture, remove excess fat and boost your beauty. Your body kinesics will be greatly improved.

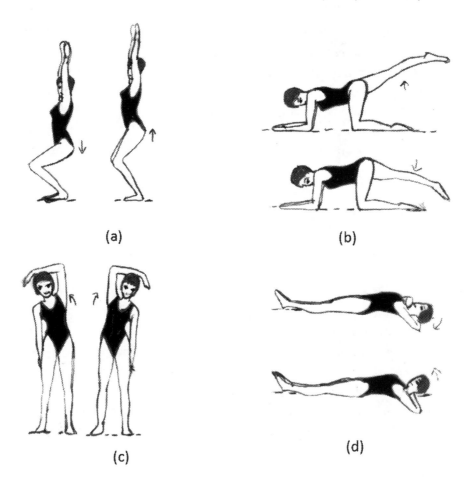

Figure 8 Toning and tightening the (a) buttock (b) thigh (c) waistline and (d) stomach muscles

9.4 REMOVE FAT AND DOUBLE CHIN LAYER

The good exercise for tones up the neck and chin is performed by turning the head to the left, then right followed by the up and down for 7 times to prevent the fat deposit around your neck and improve blood circulation. Gentle pressed using both of the left and right thumbs at the base of the neck move up in straight line below the chin before continue outward to the jaw line until base of the ears. This practice prevent double chin layer which create aging impression. Another way to prevent double chin is by holding and pressed the lower lip by the upper lip. Use thumb and index fingers of both hands to give even pressure on the back of the neck to improve the blood flow to the brain.

9.5 Tuning and Tightening Bust Shape

Aging effects due to gravity may cause the breast to fall in addition to the weak breast muscle. The beautiful breast elasticity is regain by strengthening the breast tissue using cold water compress during early morning shower or fountain water.

Another method that helps to improve the fuller breast shape is by practice uplifting exercise performed by pushing up the breasts while on laying position for eight times with 1 minutes each times. The use of breathable well supported bra from cotton fiber can reduce the sagging effect by gravity.

9.6 Cellulite

Cellulite appears in most women skin due to inactive lifestyles and poor dietary fibers. The lost of elasticity to our skin and accumulation of fat in problematic areas create uneven skin surface. The deficient nutrient for vital body's requirement can lead to sugar craving and excess sugar converted to fat combined with other fat sources create cellulite problem. The cellulite is reduced by exercising regular body stretching, aerobic, and walking to flush toxin and burn the fat deposit.

Apply circular massage on the cellulite areas with the aids of massage cream or oil to reduce cellulite problem. The simple butterfly stretching of thigh muscle in laying position while bending the knee in about 35 degree can reduce the resistant cellulite. Repeat the butterfly stretching for 7 times and proceed to the right leg stretching. To complete the exercise, continue stretching using both of the legs. Drink enough water and fibers intake to regulate and flush toxin from your body.

9.7 Flabby Arms

The arms muscle degrades with time due to repeated movement using arms forces to perform daily tasks, and routine jobs. The skin on the arms may loss elasticity quicker than other parts of our body. The arms muscle is tighten by raising the left arm up while the hand must grip weight button or any bottle. While in this position bend the elbow so that you hand can touch the back of your left shoulder do count until 7 before move your hand up and repeat the exercise for 7 times. Change the weight button to the right hand and repeated the same practice for another 7 times.

CHAPTER 10

REVELING THE HEALTHY DIET

Healthy diet must have a balance food intake according to food pyramid. Bear in mind that the optimal diet may differ from one to other individual in a population, it based on the aged, gender and physical activity. Nutrigenomics revealed the variation in human genome that is responsible for the diet varieties in a population. In reality, the composition of food consumption differs by ethnics as well as the nutrition values.

The imbalance in the nutrient intake may lead to the development of metabolic disorder diseases. The nutrient intake for early development requires lots of micronutrients and macronutrient, to ensure for healthy growth from the beginning.

The methylation of DNA leads to the epigenetic or change in the metabolic of the offspring are the result of maternal nutrition which will affect the health conditions. Choline supplement in the rat shows better memory of the offspring since choline is the precursor of the neurotransmitter acetylcholine.

10.1 ANTIOXIDANTS

The consumption of food with antioxidant compound from plant sources can fight cancer, diabetes and for rejuvenation effects. The antioxidant from varieties of fruit and vegetable are vitamins C, E and B complexes, carotenes, flavoids, isoflavoid, organo-sulphur compounds, ubiquinol, copper, manganese and magnesium. The antioxidant potential in plant species is measured in by oxygen radical absorbance capacity (ORAC), Ferric reducing antioxidant potential (FRAP) or Trolox equivalent antioxidant assay.

There are multi sources of antioxidant available from different plant species given in **Table 8**.

Table 8: Plant sources of antioxidants (Strain and Benzie, 1998)

Antioxidant	Source
Vitamin C	Blackcurrant, strawberries, kiwi fruits, citrus fruits, guava, brussel sprout, green pepper, potatoes
Vitamin E	Sweet potatoes, spinach, broccoli pulses, kale, tomato, asparagus, herb
Carotenes	Carrot, sweet potatoes, herbs, pumpkin, spinach, kale, cantaloupes, chicory, squashes, red peppers, mangoes, apricots
Lycopenes	Guavas, pink grapefruits, tomatoes
Lutein and zeaxanthin	Kale, spinach, herbs, celery, scallions, leeks
Flavonoids	Onions, strawberries, apples, citrus fruits, broad beans, peanuts, grapes, tea
Isoflavones	Pulses, soybean and linseed
Organo-sulphur compounds	Allium vegetables, garlic, onions, chives
Ubiquinol	Beans, garlic, spinach
Copper	Pulses, mushrooms, olives, guards, avocados, lychees, blackberries, blackcurrants, kiwi fruits, grapes, mangoes, guavas, bananas, raspberries, plums, asparagus, potatoes
Mangenese	Beetroot, blackberries, pineapples, pulses, spinach, bananas, raspberries

The daily consumption of Vitamin E in from natural mixed tocopherols at 200 IE, which can be blended with 100 IE of tocotrienol, the most potent cholesterol reducer. Vitamin C, a complex ascorbate is also anti-cancer with water soluble property. Wide sources of Vitamin C are available from fresh fruits. Radical scavenger of citrus origin vitamin C should be used from 500 to 1000 mg to prevent LDL cholesterol oxidation. Mixed flavonoids which can protect us from cardiovascular diseases, lung and prostate, as well as retard cancer cell should be consumed in 100 to 500 mg.

Proanthocyanidins in grape seed able to protect DNA fragmentation is required in lower dosage of 10 to 50 mg. Powerful anti-aging of resveratrol from red grape extract is taken 2 to 20 mg.

Catechin found in green tea which helps to reduce the allergic and weight loss is taken daily from 50 to 100 mg. Cranberry extract that able to decrease LDL cholesterol should be consumed in 15 to 25 mg. It is interesting fact that vitamin C applied directly on skin surface is 300 times more effective than consumed in form of liquid or tablet for skin benefit.

Consumption food with restricted calorie was found to be the most effective intervention to extent life span in mammals, as the suppression of carcinogenic effect and was linked to the conserved longevity factor (Lin, 2006).

Life journey is divided into about 5 phases from fetus to post-menopausal. Different phase require different group of nutrients. The key food requirement is highlighted in **Table 9** for different life phase (Costain, 2001).

Table 9: Key food for each phase of life

Life Phase	Key Food
Pregnancy phase for fetus and mother	Folic acid rich food from green vegetable or fortified cereals, Omega-3 sources from fish oil, rapeseed oil, pumpkin oil, walnut and wholegrain Iron-rich food, red meat, wholegrain fortified cereal, dried fruits and fish oil Calcium-rich food, milk, yogurt, cheese
Young age	Children food formula are well design in the market whereby the complete nutrient contained fortified vitamin and minerals for active growth which focus to bone and mental development
Adult	Require five portions of fruits and vegetables per day Three serving of whole grain per day Food low in saturated fat but rich in Omega-3
Elderly	Plant food with antioxidants and zinc-rich food Vitamin D from fish oil, cheese or egg Rich-fiber food from wholegrain and vegetables
Post-menopausal women	Food rich in fiber containing phytoestrogen such as soya, lentil, chick peas, pulses, bean sprouts, inseed, pumpkin seed and wholegrains Calcium-rich food like low fat milk and fortified soya foods Foods contain low saturated fat Food rich in Omega-3 and Omega-6 At least five portion of fruits and vegetables per day

A break through research on DNA damages found that DNA able to replicate 70 times for a whole life period for individual survival. In forming replication process DNA subjected to damage from free radical attack which cause mutagenic diseases (cancer) and toxic disease of inflammation. A revolutionary finding was made to find the dosage for repair the DNA by Ron Pero, using carboxyl alkyl esters (CAEs) from Cat's Claw extract.

The effectiveness of CAEs was improved further by blending with cofactor for enzyme repair of vitamin B and Zinc. The anti-aging formula was well developed using 350 mg CAEs, 100 to 300 mg niacinamide and amino acid chelated zinc of 10 to 25 mg (Giampapa et al., 2004).

Another anti-aging formula can be prepared by Coenzyme Q10 blend with ubiquinol which produce energy and prevent the oxidation of LDL cholesterol.

10.2 IMMEDIATE REMEDY FOR COMMON HEALTH PROBLEM

We are blessed with the herbs and plant species which provide natural ailments from numerous parts of the plant which contain active ingredients. The correct uses of herbs are able to treat many diseases and provide minerals and vitamins. There are 13,000 plant species with the potential use as natural medicine grown mostly in the tropic regions. The useful species for meditational cures for identified health problems were highlighted for your future uses.

1. Black fungus (*Auricularia polytricha*) is natural ailment for high blood pressure. Mushroom or fungus is well known as the food from heaven due to its fast growth cycle. A cup of black fungus is immerse into clean water overnight and bring to boil before consume the aliquot twice a day to lower the blood pressure.

2. Papaya tree leaves (*Carica papaya*) can be used to treat the hot fever from virus infection due to mosquito bites. Few papaya leaves (Figure 9) is boil in three cups of water for 5 minutes before drink a cup of the aliquot every 2 to 3 hours. The leaves and flower extract also useful for rejuvenate the body's beauty. The male flower can be used to treat excessive acidic in stomach.

3. Bitter plant or *Androghapis paniculata* is well known for reducing the blood glucose containing the active ingredient of andrographolite. A whole tree of pre-cleaned bitter plant is boiled in a milk pan for 10 minutes together with cat mustache or *Orthosiphon stamineus*. The concoction water of the shrubs species (Figure 10) shall be taken twice a day which will reduce the blood glucose level to the normal level. The usage of the concoction should not be used regularly due to its powerful ingredients. The blends can also lower the blood pressure.

4. The breast cancer can be healed by placement of bitter guard fruit juice (*Momordica charantia*) to the affected areas as well as consumption of black seed oil or black seed powder of *Nigella sativa* species.
5. Poor blood circulation and dizzy head can be healed by boiling the black beans in water with the ratio of one portion black bean to three portion of water for three hours, and used the water to improve blood circulation.

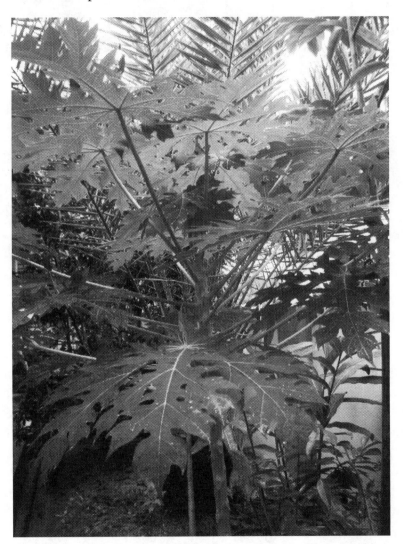

Figure 9 *Carica papaya* leaves useful for the treatment of fever and rejuvenation

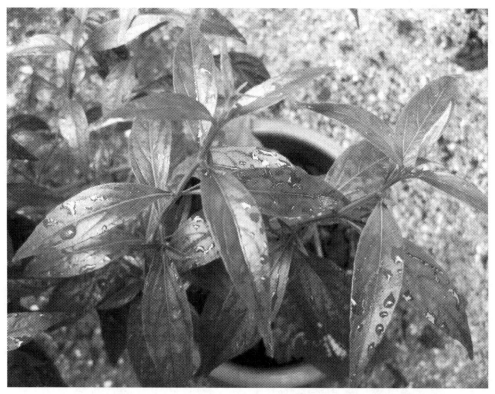

Figure 10 *Androghapis paniculata* shrubs for the treatment of diabetes mellitus

10.3 EATING FOR HEALTH

Adapting to the good eating habit, will help shaping beautiful figurine with less cholesterol and stay in lean and slim. The regular nutritional breakfast in early morning will provides energy for the whole day. The balance amount of the nutritional groups will keep body vitality where the prophet Muhammad advised to allocate our stomach into three volumes whereby one third of the stomach volume should be occupied with food, one third water and the remaining space for respiration process.

The good eating habits that improve your health and prevent diseases are:

1. The consumption of food at one time cannot be mixed up in a very complex combination, such as eating the egg should not be mixed up with fish or else if you are facing the stroke don't blame on other thing except to your own eating habit. The same advised was given by the expert for not blending the prawns and beans.

2. Do not drink immediately right after taken dinner if you want to have good body shape, wait until about 30 minutes for consume water. At night body fluid is not well regulated, it is better to drink water in form of fruits or nutritional juice.

3. When you are just finishing dishes or meal, it is not a good behavior to take a bath during that time as the stomach is in digestion process and cooling body with water will disturbed the process. Remember that what you eat will shape your body and most of the diseases started from the contaminated or incompatible food enter into your stomach.

4. If you fall sick, take breakfast early in the morning for accelerate recovery of the disease.

5. Take your meal in the sequence of fruit, protein and grain or cereal to help better digestion.

6. If you found difficult to consume certain nut or food because of it is too hard it means the food is not suitable for you.

7. Do not overload the food inside your stomach; remember that most of the diseases are started from the excessive food and bad eating habit.

8. Reduce the intake of salty food if you are approaching middle age above 40.

9. Reduce the quantity of late night meal as your body should be ready for bedtime without fully loaded with heavy food inside your stomach.

10. Those who are at risk of stroke should not consume many volatile foods which normally produce a lot of gases during digestion or the fruit with strong smell.

11. The blend of cool and hot fruit will moderate body temperature and optimize the nutrient absorption. Example of a good blend of fruit is between date and melon.

12. Reduce the consumption of junk food or processed food intake and carbonated beverages which overloaded with food additives.

Effective nutrition for body fitness was found to have close link to the intake of protein and carbohydrates. The high protein and low carbohydrate help to develop muscle and achieve weight loss. Recommended good quality of protein intake within half an hour before or after the exercise are whey proteins in 20 g per meal.

Whey protein contains amino acid, leucine that promotes the cytokine interleukin (IL-15) for anti-inflammatory, anti-obesity, muscle-regenerating signaling agent that activated the longevity gene of SIRT-1. The minimum leucine dosage for body maintenance is 1 to 3 g per day. Numerous sources of leucine can be found in beef, chicken, egg, milk, salmon, cheese, chick peas and almond.

Fasting is good practice for stay young as the empty stomach help to lower metabolic system. Periodic fasting alternate with exercise generate acute oxidative stress that keeps mitochondria, neuro-motors and fiber stay intact. Acute oxidative stress helps muscle increase resilient to the oxidative stress simultaneously promote the glutathione and superoxide dismutases (SOD) production while optimize the use of energy (Ori Hofmekler) to eliminate reactive oxygen species (ROS).

Excessive ROS will contribute to the cell membrane damage, DNA mutations, CVD, atherosclerosis, cancer, diabetes, neurodegenerative diseases, inflammation, emphysema, cataracts, toxicity and vitamin deficiency (Wu and Cederbaum, 2015).

Controlling the food intake seem to be the best and convenient approach to provide healthy body well-being as less calories food is better way to reverse aging but not a popular method to food industry (Winkler, 1998).

Fruit juices prepared from fresh fruit not only rich in antioxidant but also provide benefit to your body. **Table 10** shows good blend of fruit juices that can prepared at home and benefit for your body.

Table 10 Healthy fruit juice blends for body improvement

Fruit juices	Benefit
Carrot, ginger and apple	Boost and clean the stomach
Apple, cucumber and celery	Prevent cancer, reduce cholesterol
Tomato, carrot and apple	Improve skin complexion and eliminate bad breadth
Bitter guard, apple and milk	Avoid bad breadth and reduce internal body heat
Orange, ginger and cucumber	Improve skin texture, moisturize and reduce body heat
Pineapple, apple and water melon	Dispel excess salt, nourishes the bladder and kidney
Apple, cucumber and kiwifruit	Improve skin complexion
Pear and banana	Regulates sugar content
Carrot, apple, pear and mango	Reduce body heat, counteract toxin, decreased blood pressure and fight oxidization
Honeydew, grape, water melon and milk	Increase cell activity and strengthen body immunity
Banana, pineapples and milk	Rich in nutritious and prevent constipation

CHAPTER 11
VITAL ORGAN FOR BEAUTIFUL BLOSSOM

11.1 KIDNEY FOR LIQUIDITY FILTRATION

The kidney helps regulate the water content of the blood by filtering about half a cup body fluid each minute where the water is reabsorbed into the blood by passive osmosis controlled by vasopressin. During extremely dry season body face dehydration with affect water loss, increase blood concentration with less blood volume causing body to induce more vasopressin to minimize water loss. Kidney damage occurs when exposed to toxic substances such as arsenic, mercury, organic compounds, insecticides, microorganisms. The only option for patients with chronic kidney disease (CKD) is to use hemodialysis to purify the blood in a regular period.

The kidney failure occurs when Glomeruler filtration rate (GFR) of affected person was found at 15 ml/min or below. The affected person with CKD is advised to consume low protein diet and take keto acid treatment. People with diabetic, hypertension and arthritis are more prone to have CKD. Other factors such as obesity, aged groups above 60 years, regular consumption of painkiller or have family history with CKD are at higher risk of facing CKD.

11.2 LIVER FOR ALL THE GOOD SENSES

The most important organ in human body is liver which carry the function to detoxify toxin and metabolize drug in our blood. Liver is the largest internal organ responsible for regulate the insulin for controlling blood sugar. The organ itself is subjected to the viral attack and may be saturated with fat molecules in forms of bad cholesterol. Liver damage from hepatitis occurs in silent infected from the host career in human being.

Liver diseases like hepatitis A, B and C are affected by viruses. Cirrhosis or jaundice also related to the liver diseases. Liver cancer developed in liver cell is known as hepatocellular carcinoma while metastatic cancer is form from nearby affected organ.

Practice liver cleansing for removing accumulate toxin at least twice a year using liver flush blends containing grapefruit, lemon, olive oil and garlic. Consume liver food diet weekly containing leafy green and cruciferous vegetables, grapefruit, lemon and lime, beet, carrot, avocado, apples, walnut, cabbage, turmeric and olive oil.

11.3 HEART THE KEY FOR LIFE SURVIVOR

The heart functions as life machine to ensure the fresh oxygen enter into the lung cavity and regulate oxygenized blood flow to the whole body. Animal species also depend on the oxygen to carry metabolic reaction in a complex conversion system with slight modification for different medium. The inhale contaminated air into respiratory system may deposit toxic compounds on the lung surface form hardened scar which inhibit it function and cause cancer in long term exposure.

Other potential risk is fat accumulation on the arteries wall which may constrict the blood flow. The cardiovascular disease associated with the heart failure is one of leading cause of death. The coronary heart disease, stroke and heart attack are the common disease in modern world. The prevention of cardiovascular disease may well relate to the consumption of food containing low trans-fatty acid from processed food, fried food and margarine.

Food containing trans-fatty acid increases the cytokines and total cholesterol in our body. Low-density lipoprotein (LDL) and high-density lipoprotein (HDL) forms total cholesterol but only HDL is favorable since the LDL may attribute to the formation of clogged arteries. The normal level of LDL and HDL are <2.6 mmol/L and >1.04 mmol/L accordingly.

Cholesterol intake is minimize by changing in cooking techniques from deep frying to steaming, boiling and grilling, or used healthier ingredient in preparation of meal which contain less fat and oil.

The heart health supplements are:

1. Minerals of calcium, chromium and magnesium
2. Bioflavonoids of carotenes such as bilberry
3. EPA and DHA from fish oil
4. Alpha linolenic acid from flaxseed

5. Gingko biloba herbs
6. Inulin, psyllium husk, soy and citrus fibers
7. Lecithin phospholipid
8. Cholestatins from plant sterols
9. Vitamin A, C and E
10. High amylose starches

CHAPTER 12
SYNERGIZING THE BODY'S ENERGY

12.1 ENERGY HOUSE

Human body requires enough energy to perform daily activities and metabolic function. The energy source comes from four energy houses found in human body. The first energy is located at the center of body's matrix. Assemble from the origins of life formation in the fetus development which feed by this center. Similarly a grown up man may find their energy from their belly. Toning the belly muscle will increase the inner power while maintain the healthy states and control the respiration system. In fact, if you refer to Yoga practice, most of the workouts begin with the alignment of your hand to the center of body which can strengthen the muscle and intensify the force. While in Muslim's prayer, the most significant position is in standing posture and holding both hands close to the belly.

The generated and stored energy may be reduced by the deposit of fat around the belly which blocks the flow of energy. Those who have round shapes where the weight is center around the belly are more prone to many diseases this includes heart attack, kidney failure and diabetes.

12.2 MENTAL ENERGY

The energy in the brain moves from the brain cell to the outer universe in form of waves and travel through the air to the expected target. Synergizing the mental energy means focusing to the personal objectives which can act as magnet toward visualize matters. The mind block occurs due to unconnected synapse to carry the memory or intended functions. The synapses use to transmit the signal between neuron cell in form of rapid impulse from axon-axon, axon-dendrite or dendrite-dendrite. A neuron cell is fires from 5-50 times per second. The vital nutrient for the brain must be available to regenerate brain cell.

Quite interesting fact is that those who use to be very talkative can cause the brain to shrink more compare to those who talk less. The noticeable effects of this shrink are quite similar to the face where more wrinkle and face lines can be observed especially at old ages. Brain cell capacity can be enhanced while aging process by activate more connection in the neuron cell even though it was believes that memory loss increase at old age causing damage in the cell due to the affected diseases, which reduce the body responses in performing physical activity.

Memory loss or amnesia is related to the brain damage in the hippocampus area that used to encode, store and retrieve the memory. Regular brain exercise is one of the ways to fight the aging process. Provide challenge to the mind by playing Sudoku, learning new language or create new hobby. Remember during young age, the brain capability is developed by exposing to new challenges and learning new things, so in summary don't stop learning. It was found by the scientist that individuals with O blood carry more grey cells than individual with other blood groups. And the grey cell improve the mental capability and functionally better that the other brain cell.

Neuron in the brain is continuing to replenish while aging take place. The brain degenerative effect of Alzheimer's disease may be experienced by 1 out of 10 of aged population above 65 years old. It was found that the Alzheimer's disease is caused by beta-amyloid plaques from protein fragment occupying spaces in the afflicted brain nerve cell and neurofibrillary tangles in the neurons. The effect of Alzheimer's disease of loss of cognitive skill and confusion require caretaker for the patients which treated by temporary drug.

Mental energy is drive by the type of food intake which may influence the way how people made decision, acceptance in spiritual believes and conceptual theory versus reality and reflects common behavior during socializing. Human civilizations developed by the acceptable ethic shown as per individual response toward himself and other peoples need in a manner that adjusted to the mental wellbeing of the whole population.

The best food for improve brain memory and cognitive skill are honey blend with ginger juice (*Zingiber officinale*) and saffron (*Crocus sativus*). Other useful food for brain are lentils, black seeds, cloves, frankincense and raisins in the diets can sharpen the mental capability and promote learning acuity.

12.2.1 Brain waves

Our brain waves are the electrical waves in the brain cell that characterized by the level of consciousness where the wave pattern is classified into beta, alpha, theta and delta. Each pattern has different wave lengths that indicate the state of mind adapted to their environment for performing different types of activities. The brain waves can be activated by listening to the music which can induced the specific wave, especially for inculcate the learning capability, achieving target or objective in combination with mental framing or affirmation. This method was used to accelerate intended wishes or aims in personal life, career or life. Utilizing the brain as powerful energy to attract materials also referred to the law of attraction which was successfully utilized by few who put into believes of the law. The waves have specific range and function as follows:

The beta waves in 13-30 Hz are conducive for learning and applied logical, analytical, intellectual thinking and verbal communication. Beta states of mind remain active during working time and help to reduce fatigue. Waves higher than 30 to 35 affect the nervous system and all negatives thought occur in this range. The higher frequencies of more than 30 Hz are known as gamma waves.

The alpha waves in 8-12 Hz are applicable for creative problem solving, accelerated learning, and suitable for stress and anxiety reduction, inspiration and motivation. Alpha state is used to promote relaxation, memory improvement and induce reflection. The alpha range is stimulated by deep relaxation, simulation of pineal gland in the brain and meditation. The pineal gland is activated by the Yoga breathing exercises through rhythmic breathing and alternate nostril breathing.

Theta waves in 4-7 Hz are conducive for profound inner peace, suitable for physical and emotional healing. The wave is achieved during meditation or light sleep which can improve physic abilities and retrieve unconscious experience or material as well as reduce anxiety.

Delta waves in 5-4 Hz are slowest waves in deep sleep condition promote healing of headaches, reduce anxiety, divine knowledge, personal growth, trauma recovery and can connected to the universe's facts and figures.

12.2.2 Brain booster

The brain can be energized by taking equal amount of herbs consists of peppermint, Siberian ginseng, skull cap, wood betony, gotu-kola and kelp in forms of capsule or tea pack. Oat consumption can strengthen and fortify the nerve system while licorice can improve the memory. The other ways to improve the brain is by wearing green or blue beryl, red ruby and pearl gemstones for a smarter state of mind.

12.3 HEART ENERGY

Relationship of your heart to the mind is like flowing water and river bank. The energy is connected to the mind dramatically enhance by visualization or senses. Heart energy is magnified by abstract factors such as love, care or concern. Even the emotion detected by the brain cell located at the base of brain center connected directly to the heart may play a big role in human health through psychological behavior or auto body response. The heart energy can help body self-healing and create extraordinary strength for fighting with deadly diseases like cancer or dangerous situation. The example of the heart energy overrule the mind energy can be seen in the case of an attempt by a mother to rescue her son during fires accidents even though knowing that she may face fatally. The drive of the mother's action is totally due to the heart energy, the love.

12.4 GEN 2 ENERGY

The last energy resource is used for sustainability and survival. The energy ensures the continuous generation of population located below the stomach. Practically the energy is actively used by the young and middle age groups whose stay active in their sexual lives. In facts, the overused of this energy can shorten the life span. The Gen 2 energy easily reduces due to lacks of nutrient or health care, or poor lifestyles, contamination from toxic substances. The block of this energy sector will weaken the reproductive capacity and the diabetic conditions, high blood pressure and heart disease may have adverse effect to this energy. The energy in this house can be increased using a bitter plants species which improve the fire elements in our body.

All of the energy sources can feed to all the seven energy storages or chakras to activate whole body functions. Remember that the energy may be absorbed by negative entity from the environment similar like draining energy from a battery pack. It is important to create the shield of protection layer to prevent ones body's energy been robbed by such negative entity. Shielding effect for protection can be simulated by mind visualization or imagination of the silver layer around your body during early morning meditation or after prayer.

Correct energy state is a must for a healthier body to carry its metabolic functions and protect from many diseases and infections. The symptom of low energy is reflected by the fatigue body and confusion. This will affect your judgments in giving out spontaneous response and decision makings, the best thing to do is take a good rest to recharge your energy by having a deep sleep or eat healthy meal if you are in empty stomach and removes all of the negatives energy trapped inside your body by the following the steps given under stress relieves method and de-stress activity.

REFERENCES

Azahari Ibrahim (2000) Ubat-ubatan Tradisional Arab-Melayu Penawar 200 Penyakit Kuala Lumpur, Darul Nu'man.

Aida Osman (1997) Gemuk, antara kesihatan dan penampilan diri, Utusan Malaysia, 25 July 1997

Asiah Mon (1997) Aromaterapi - rawatan menggunakan pati minyak, Utusan Malaysia, 8 Ogos 1997

Clare Maxwell-Hudson's (1994) Aromatherapy Massage Book, Dorling Kindersley Limited, U.K.

Constain, L. (2001) Super Nutrients Handbook. London, Dorling Kindersley Limited.

Daar, A.S., Singer, P.A.,Persad, D.L., Pramming, S.K.,Matthews, A.R., Beaglehole, R., Bernstein, A., Borysiewicz, L.K., Abdallah, S., Ganguly, N., Glass, R.I., Finegood, D.T., Kopla, J.,Nabel, E.G., Sarna, G.,Sarrafzadegan, N., Smith, R., Yach, D. and Bell. J. (2007). Grand challenges in chronic non-communicable diseases. Nature 450, 494-496.

Dayle Had Don (1999) Ageless Beauty -A women guide to lifelong beauty and well-being, Aurum Press. U.K.

Desai, T.P. (1999). Stress and mental workload: A conceptual synthesis. In D.M. Pestonjee, U. Pareek & R. Aggarwal (Eds.) Studies in Stress and its Management. Pp. 47-90. New Delhi, Oxford & IBH Publishing

Dr. Rajeev Sharma, Water Therapy, Goodwill Publishing House, India.

Edward C. Geehr (2008) Does Vitamin D Prevent Breast Cancer.

Erasmus, U. (2003). Fats that heal and fats that kill, Oak Publication PJ, Malaysia.

Eskay Shazryl and Jarrod Hanks (1994).Sport and stress therapy. Eskay Inc. USA.

George D. Pamplona-Roger (2002). Diet Penyembuh Ajaib, Editorial Safeliz, S.L.

Georgette Mosbacher (1993) Feminine Force, release the power within to create the life you deserve. Simon & Schuster, N.Y.

Giampapa, V., Pero, R. & Zimmerman, M. (2004). The Anti Aging Solution. New Jersey, John Wiley & Sons.

Griffith, H. Winter (1989) Complete Guide to Pediatric Symptom, Illness & Medications, The Body Press.

Gruenemay, J. (2005).Calculating your daily calorific need. Lifescript

Guariguata, L, Whiting, D. R., Hambleton, I. Beagley, J., Linnenkamp, U. and Shaw, J.E. (2014) Global estimates of diabetes prevalence for 2013 and projections for 2035, *Diabetes Res. Clin. Pract.,* vol. 103, pp. 137-149.

JVC-7 (2003). Seventh report of the joint national committee on prevention, detection, evaluation, and treatment of high blood pressure, American Heart Association, Inc.

Jane Plant (2014). Your life is in your hands. St Martin Press, Thomas Dune Books

Judith Lazarus (2000) Stress Relief & Relaxation Techniques, McGraw Hill.

Letha Hadady (2003). Healthy Beauty using nature's secrets to look great and feel terrific. New Jersey, John Wiley & Sons, Inc.

Lin, Su-Ju (2009). Molecular mechanisms of longevity regulation and calorie restriction. In James Kaput & Raymond L. Rodriguez (Eds.) Nutritional Genomics. Pp. 207-218. New Jersey, John Wiley & Sons.

Mark Evens (2004). Tranform your mind, body and spirit. London, Southwater, Annes Publishing Ltd.

Moashing Ni (2009). Decode your tongue. LiftScript, 29 March 2015

MOH (2014). Management Guidelines of Malaria in Malaysia, Vector Borne Disease Sector, Disease Control Division Ministry of Health Malaysia

Moss Greene (2015). Food calorie chart of healthy foods to lose weight. http://CommonSenseHealth. com/food-calorie-chart-of-healthy-foods-to-lose-weight. 25 May 2015

Ngau Heong Tabib China (2002). Kaedah Terapi Urut Guasa Traditional China. Johore Bahru, Syarikat Percetakan Taley.

NIH -National Institute of Health (2015). Calculate Your Body and Mass Index, http://www.nhlbi. nih.gov/health/educational. 23 Mac 2015

Paul Galbraith (1998) Reverse Ageing the natural way, Thorson, U.K.

Peter Chin Kean Choy, t'ai-chi chi kung - fifteen ways to a happier you. Rainbow T'ai-Chi Chi Kung Centre

Raflas Sabirin (2011) Pengubatan Al-Quran Penawar Segala Penyakit, mmp communication Sdn. Bhd.

Sabika Zehra Zaidi and Naima K Gulrez (2006) Stress and Obesity A killer Relationship. In Akbar Husain and Mohd Ilyas Khan, Recent Trend in Human Stress Management. Pp.192-199. India, Global Vision Publishing House.

Stay Well Magazine, Mitochondria cell. July 2014

Strain J.J & Benzie, I.F.F. (1998) Antioxidant nutrients. In Michele J. Sadler and Michael Saltmarsh (Eds.) Functional Foods the Consumer, the Products and the Evidence. Pp. 74-79. Cambridge, UK, The Royal Society of Chemistry

Susan L. Levy, Carol Lehr (1996) Your body can talk, how to use simple muscle testing to learn what your body knows and needs, Hohm Press.

UNAIDS (2011) World aids day report: How to get to zero: faster, smarter, better, JC2216E

Vernon Coleman (2006) Bodypower The secret of self-healing. Masterpiece Publication.

Vernon Coleman (2001) How to live longer and stay young for the rest of your life. Masterpiece Publication.

Winkler, J.T. (1998) The Future of Functional Food. In Michele J. Sadler and Michael Saltmarsh (Eds.) Functional Foods the Consumer, the Products and the Evidence. Pp. 74-79. Cambridge, UK, The Royal Society of Chemistry

Wu, D and Cederbaum, A.I (2015) Alcohol, Oxidative Stress and Free Radical Damage, National Institute on Alcohol Abuse and Alcoholism, U.S. http://pubs.niaaa.nih.gov/publications/arh27-4/277-284.htm. 25 July 2015.

Modern lifestyle exposed many health threats to the population through rapid changes in technology and new materials designated to meet the market demand. This will change how people's work, socialize and adapt to the environment. Complex life challenge has leads to stress development, new disease outbreak and infection. The knowledge on healthy diet, balance nutrient, health care and fitness practices are vital for all. Discover simple techniques and tips on de-stress, counter ageing effect and toning your muscles for the healthier body while gaining the lean shape. Protect your body from physical and mental health risks, and reduce the affected diseases by natural way not only improve life but also save your spending on medicine and consultation fees.

The health is your genuine wealth and the beauty
is signature of healthy body - A.M. Zain

'Experience is your best teacher'

The tougher the experiences, the better you develop solving skills capability.

A. M. Zain is very dedicated in taking care of her health and beauty. The efforts bear fruitful results at the end of the day, lead her live free from prescribe medicines or medical bills. This book share her thought on how to stay in good shape through simple body fitness practices, balance diet, stay away from infections and diseases naturally, while improve mind, body contour, toning and uplift muscles through numerous of techniques.

Printed in the United States
By Bookmasters